AF371454

COMPUTERIZED MEDICAL DIAGNOSIS:

A NOVEL SOLUTION TO AN OLD PROBLEM

Carlos Feder   **2006**

For the diagnostic algorithm, a patent is pending

ISBN 0-7414-3593-4

Published by:

INFINITY
PUBLISHING.COM

1094 New Dehaven Street, Suite 100
West Conshohocken, PA 19428-2713
Info@buybooksontheweb.com
www.buybooksontheweb.com
Toll-free (877) BUY BOOK
Local Phone (610) 941-9999
Fax (610) 941-9959

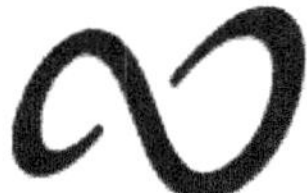

Printed in the United States of America
Printed on Recycled Paper
Published December 2006

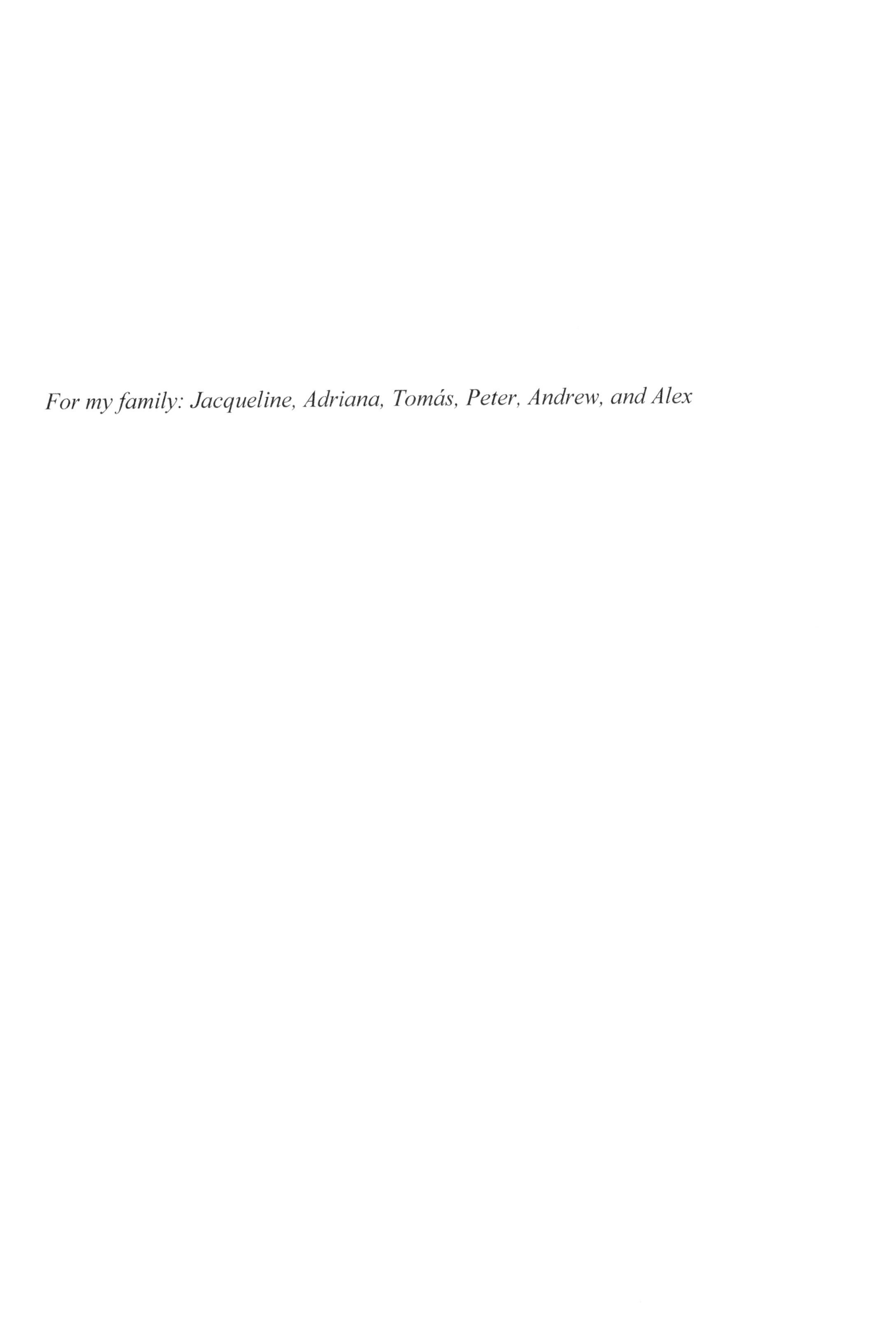

For my family: Jacqueline, Adriana, Tomás, Peter, Andrew, and Alex

ACKNOWLEDGEMENTS

My appreciation goes back to my Argentinean friends and colleagues, who helped me get the grants that encouraged me to more seriously pursue my research on computerized medical diagnosis. I especially remember Manuel Luis Martí, Julio Andrés Belomo, and Raúl de los Santos; forgive me if after so many years I forgot somebody.

My son Tomás was always by my side, helping me with his extraordinary gifts for mathematics and theoretical computation. His imaginative and original contributions greatly facilitated my research.

To my wife Jacqueline, I owe uncountable hours of support and patience, while I sat before my computer, deeply submerged in thought.

Special thanks go to my friend John Reiland, a Renaissance man with a vast knowledge about many different subjects. He is an excellent scientific writer with knowledge of medicine that surpasses some physicians. He spent uncountable hours editing my book without accepting any financial retribution. He must not be blamed for the many grammatical and literary errors that still remain, because we had insufficient time to complete his meticulous job. Medicine is plagued with semantic problems that triggered serious fights with my editor, ending with reconciliation and valuable clarification of important concepts.

CONTENTS

INTRODUCTION

This book is organized in several parts.

The **first part**, a short autobiography, presents some of my background that is relevant to the subject of this research.

The **second part** highlights the paramount importance of computerized diagnosis to patients, physicians, and essentially all medically related organizations. During recent years it seems as if interest in computerized diagnostic programs has declined in favor of other research goals.

Some of these goals pursued in the academic field are concerned with abstracting formal representations of knowledge (*ontologies* [1]) from a specific domain or instantiation, to be applied or reused within other domains (*e.g.*, PROTÉGÉ program [2].) Considerable effort has been dedicated to timing of medical events (*e.g.*, RESUMÉ program [3] [4]), syntactic and semantic aspects of medical knowledge and language (*e.g.*, SNOMED), creation of guidelines for management of diseases (*e.g.*, GLIF [5] [6], SAGE [7]), medical informatics and the Internet [8], etc. Other goals are financially oriented, such as billing, coding, and administrative programs for hospitals and private offices, storage of medical information in hand held devices, and others.

This change of motivations has been called "the winter of computerized diagnosis" and could be ascribed in part to frustration encountered while attempting to create a diagnostic program. I am trying to bring a new spring to this subject.

The **third part** defines medical concepts and terminology such as health and disease, clinical data, syndrome, diagnosis, among others. This primarily is intended for non-medical specialists such as computer scientists, mathematicians, statisticians, and programmers. It also may be useful for medical students or recent graduates who have experienced the fragmentation of medicine into subjects such as pathology, pathogenesis, pathophysiology, and internal medicine, and have not yet had an opportunity to integrate all of them into the whole picture of medicine; they see the trees but not the forest.

The **fourth part** discloses the principles on which our diagnostic program is based, analyzing past errors that hindered the creation of a satisfactory algorithm. Essential requirements for such a program are enumerated; they are not gathered in a specific chapter, but are interspersed, where pertinent, in the general text.

The **fifth part** describes how our diagnostic program operates. Ideas that facilitate the conversion of medical reasoning into a practical algorithm are explained. This parallelism between human clinical reasoning and a computerized algorithm is useful not only for creation of a computerized diagnostic program, but also to acquaint medical students with the process of clinical reasoning.

Appendix A summarizes the integration of our medical knowledge base and diagnostic algorithm, also shown in flowchart format. Our diagnostic algorithm comprises novel concepts that are expected to make possible the creation of an efficient and accurate diagnostic program able to perform at a medical specialist level. Patent is pending.

Appendix B discloses basic aspects of the user interface.

SHORT AUTOBIOGRAPHY RELATED TO COMPUTER DIAGNOSIS

I am Carlos Feder. I was born in Vienna, Austria in 1929. At age five, my mother dragged my father and me to Trieste, Italy, seeking better living conditions. After one unsuccessful year, we moved to Paris, France; three years later, when I was nine years old, we immigrated to Argentina. My mother's nomadic and restless spirit did not make us wealthy, but unforeseeably saved us from the Nazi holocaust. I attended the University of Buenos Aires Medical School, graduating in 1954. I completed my internship and residency at the same institution. In addition to managing a busy private practice for 30 years, I taught internal medicine for 20 years at the university hospital. In Argentina, I met my wife Jacqueline, who, apart from making my life enjoyable, gave me the present of our two children, Adriana and Tomás.

I am telling this story not only to relate my background but also to apologize for any literary flaws that this publication may have, because English is not my first language, but my fifth.

Due to poor memory, I had difficulty remembering the myriad of diseases and their corresponding symptoms, signs, tests, and procedures—I had to work twice as hard to equal my colleagues. This deficiency motivated me to consider using a computer for this task. At that time, this was a completely original idea, at least in Argentina. This was prior to the advent of personal computers. Available computers were uncommon, very expensive, filled entire rooms, and required powerful ventilation systems to remove the heat generated by a multitude of vacuum tubes. My plan was to make these computers available at specialized medical centers, where they could be used for diagnosing difficult cases.

The effort involved in starting a new medical practice distracted me from this project. Another negative quality, my obsessive-compulsive trait (not quite a disorder) constantly brought me back to my computerized diagnosis obsession.

At the University of Buenos Aires, to become a professor of internal medicine, one had to complete a six-year postgraduate career that included some extracurricular courses such as Philosophy, History of Science, History of Medicine, and Methodology of Science and Research, among others, each requiring submission of a corresponding term paper. For my Methodology of Science and Research course in 1964, I chose the topic "Cybernetic Clinic," in which I initially expressed my ideas about how to approach computer assisted diagnosis.

In 1980, while visiting the United States, I saw in a shop window a strange device that resembled a typewriter with a keyboard but without type bars. That happened to be the first Apple personal computer. I immediately purchased this fascinating invention and took it to Argentina. Upon my return, I played with my new toy and experimented with programming in Basic. All this was done with the help of my very bright son Tomás, at that time age 15.

I demonstrated my new computer and its potential for medical applications at lectures for physicians in the Department of Medicine. I became known for my obsession with this subject. One day, the head of the department asked me to publish a paper about computer-assisted diagnosis in an important medical journal, "La Semana Médica," which I did in 1980 [9].

Finally, Roemmers pharmaceutical company gave me a grant of US$ 20,000 to further explore the possibility of creating a computerized medical diagnostic program. This amount—at that time considerable by Argentinean standards—enabled me to focus more intently on the problem. I traveled several times to the United States to consult with experts, search the medical computer literature, and learn the latest technological advances. I was fortunate to meet my distinguished colleagues Ted Shortliffe, Harold Sox, and Mark Perlroth at Stanford, and Marsden Blois and Dana Ludwig at UCSF. All were kind to my then 17 year old son and me, spending considerable time sharing their knowledge and experience. They provided me with bibliographic references. I visited medical libraries, copied numerous papers, and bought books, which I took to Buenos Aires, for my research. With part of the grant money I bought a very heavy and noisy Corvus external hard disk with a "fabulous" capacity of 10 MB, for $6,000 (a bargain at that time.) My unfortunate wife had difficulty sleeping when I was working in an adjacent room in the middle of the night.

In September 1983, after many long years of struggling to immigrate to the United States, I finally obtained USA residence for my family and my medical license for California. Both of my children were admitted to Stanford University. These events were the turning points that finally convinced my reluctant wife to agree to the fulfillment of my American dream. One of my objectives was to pursue my computer research in this new country. After an unsuccessful attempt to interest venture capitalists in my project, I again had to struggle to build up from scratch a new existence. It took several years to achieve financial stability in my solo medical practice in Palo Alto, California, which then absorbed all of my time and energy for the next 19 years. But my latent obsession remained; it occasionally surfaced in the form of a new idea.

Eventually, at age 72, after half a century of full dedication to my medical practice I elected to retire on January 1, 2002. And guess what? I finally was free to dedicate time at leisure to my long-battered project. What puzzled me most at that time, was that the problem of computerized diagnosis was not yet satisfactorily solved, after more than 50 years of endeavor. This was difficult to explain considering the fabulous progress of computer technology with processor's tremendous speed of gigaherz and hard discs of many gigabytes, accessible at low price on one hand, and the existence of privileged human brains all over the world on the other.

The reasons perhaps are twofold: either the project is not feasible because human diagnostic skills are too complex to be emulated by computer programs, or something is wrong in the approach to the problem. I decided to dedicate one full year to attempt to discover which premise is correct; intuition told me the latter was correct. I based this gut feeling on my third mental weakness, the first being my bad memory; the second, my obsessive trait; and the third, my conviction that I am not a genius. I consider myself to possess only an average intellectual capacity. Nevertheless, I still proved to be a good physician during my 50 years of practice, typically arriving at correct diagnoses; at least this was confirmed by positive feedback that I received from my patients and colleagues. If only average intelligence is required to achieve a diagnosis, then the diagnostic process could hardly be so complicated that it would be impossible to convert it to a computer algorithm.

Because I was able to dedicate more time to the problem, my efforts were rewarded. Suspecting that we researchers base our search on prior studies that to me often seemed incorrect, I decided to ignore all published ideas and approach the problem from scratch. Introspection and analysis of my own diagnostic psychology uncovered several new findings and clarified some errors committed by other researchers and myself.

In the following chapters, I will discuss what I consider methodological errors that hindered the development of a successful computerized medical diagnosis program, and define the requirements for a workable program. The algorithm that I developed must be tested with a prototype program to dispel uncertainties and correct imperfections, before implementing a final version.

Publishing a study without an updated bibliography generally is considered unacceptable. Because my prior literature search ended around 1983, I needed to correct this deficiency; this involved becoming acquainted with newer computer diagnostic programs such as ILIAD [10], QMR [11] [12], GIDEON, and DXplain. While analyzing these programs I noticed that some of my ideas had already been described. However, my research includes observations and principles not found in the literature, and that are sufficiently original to justify publication and facilitate the creation of a more efficient computer diagnostic program.

THE IMPORTANCE OF A COMPUTER DIAGNOSTIC PROGRAM

Treatment errors and its consequences are widely published in medical literature and by public media. Diagnostic errors are less publicized, perhaps because they are less apparent, poorly recognized and admitted by committing physicians. However, these errors are detected by consultants or other colleagues who inhered the patient. Some diagnostic errors are inconsequential, thanks to Mother Nature that facilitates spontaneous cure despite the physician, but others may lead to serous disability and demise.

Non-computerized diagnosis requires that clinicians remember several thousand currently known diseases with their corresponding names, symptoms, causes, mechanisms, and so forth. Diseases not recalled or never learned would not be diagnosed.

Considering the explosive growth of medical knowledge, it is impossible to memorize everything. This serious problem has been relieved in part with the advent of medical specialists. Each specialty deals only with a specific segment of the medical knowledge referring to a certain organ, body system, or class of causes (*e.g.*, dermatology, gastroenterology, neurology, infectious diseases, oncology.) However, the medical knowledge is becoming so vast that even a specialist no longer can remember all requisite facts, resulting in the creation of subspecialties. This solution is imperfect, producing communication problems among subspecialists, specialists, and the primary care physician. Patient care also is partitioned among these different physicians. Specialists are not always readily available, especially in rural settings. Because of time constraints, medical emergencies often do not allow specialist consultations; the attending physician may have to make a vital decision based on partial and incomplete knowledge. For these reasons, implementation of computer diagnosis is of paramount importance.

Computers can be of great assistance in such situations. With their tremendous memory capacity, they can readily store the contents of many medical texts. Their processors can rapidly retrieve the needed information anywhere and at any time. For diagnosis in general, an efficient diagnostic program could likely even replace specialists.

A diagnostic program can be expanded to retrieve pertinent prognostic and therapeutic information.

Why, if computerized medical diagnostic is so important, no practical program to assist physicians at the bedside of a patient has been achieved after more than half a century of endeavor? Reasons are manifold:

- The problem is interdisciplinary; computer scientists do not posses the experience of seasoned internists, familiar with daily nuances of medical practice; physicians in general lack the mathematical and logical skills that computer science requires. This incongruity led to the creation of diagnostic programs that at best only are used for diagnostic training, but inadequate to elucidate patient's current ailment. The present publication, in addition to discuss novel ideas to achieve success in this field, has the intention to provide a kind of textbook with the basics in diagnostic medicine and also to illustrate computational aspects of a workable diagnostic algorithm.

- Inherent difficulty of the task; medicine has many aspects that are difficult to translate into computer algorithms.

- The erroneous belief that the many nuances of daily medical practice can be represented by sometimes sophisticated mathematical tools, totally divorced from clinical reality.

- Misuse of Bayes formula or other probabilistic tools in some existing algorithms.

- Algorithms based on inexact premises.

- Some loss of interest or patience of researchers, distracted by other more tangible projects related to the medical establishment. Time is overdue to return to the drawing board and devise a computer program that is concordant with human diagnostic reasoning and practice, objective of this book.

Existing diagnostic programs, some commercially available, typically offer only limited diagnostic information. When patient's symptoms (we call them *clinical data*) are provided to the computer, these programs typically retrieve a long list of possible diagnoses, instead of pinpointing more specifically one or a few; most exclude very rare diseases. The calculation of the probability of each of such diagnoses is usually inaccurate, because it typically relies on Bayes formula, which in my opinion is inadequate for this purpose. Bayes calculation requires that clinical data manifested by a patient be independent and exhaustive, and diagnoses be incompatible, conditions that are not fulfilled by internal medicine and actual clinical cases. Few of these programs, if any, recommend the *probabilistically calculated* best cost-benefit clinical datum to investigate in the patient at each diagnostic step, to achieve more efficiently, economically, and sooner a final diagnosis. None recommends, on a probabilistically calculated base, a *set* of clinical data to be investigated simultaneously in the patient. This is essential in emergency situations, but also important in an outpatient stetting, to avoid the need of the physician to contact the patient after each single new test result to order the next one. This best choice function eliminates the request of many unnecessary tests, which is extremely important in this era of managed care, in which medical insurers are pressuring physicians to reduce expenses; on the other hand it will preclude curtailing really necessary tests or procedures. It also would protect physicians from unjustified malpractice suits; if the computer program is flawless and universally respected, its recommendations will become standard of care. Cost of investigating a clinical datum is mentioned by some authors. Our algorithm interprets cost not only as dollar expense, but also includes discomfort and risk of the procedure; it uses a novel method of qualitatively estimating these three elements and *considering the greatest of such elements as equal to the overall cost*. Neither do other programs typically diagnose *concurrent diseases* afflicting simultaneously a specific patient or *complex clinical presentations* of a specific disease with its diverse complications and associations of clinical entities. *Interactions between concurrent diseases or drugs that may mask important clinical data* of the primary disease, and many other nuances related to clinical practice are not considered. Our algorithm addresses all these unsolved problems.

Such an algorithm, if successful in medicine, may represent a more general model of reasoning; a paradigm of mental structure and functioning applicable to other inexact disciplines such as law, sociology, politics, defense, or corporate strategy.

MEDICAL CONCEPTS AND TERMINOLOGY

Some confusion and a lack of consensus exist concerning medical terminology; definitions provided by medical dictionaries often are incomplete or incorrect. The terminology used in this publication represents a compromise among current usage, personal experience, and applicability to our computer algorithm.

HEALTH AND DISEASE

In medical school, the human being is revealed as a very complex physicochemical system in which many unceasing reactions maintain physiological constants within a prescribed range of values. This essence of life is shared with all other living organisms. We leave to the reader how he wants to fill in this rather materialistic definition according to his or her spiritual or religious belief, but from a practical didactic and computational perspective, the given definition is convenient and acceptable.

To define **health** or its related concept of **normality** is more difficult than it might appear. Some use a statistical concept: if a person's physicochemical parameter values (*e.g.*, body temperature, heart rate, blood glucose) remain within the range of those of the majority of the population, he or she is considered normal or healthy. Others associate health with a subjective feeling of well-being, harmonious bodily functions, and an ability to establish and fulfill one's goals in life. These definitions are complementary.

Disease is the opposite of health: a condition in which some physicochemical parameter values are out of range and health qualities are impaired, typically resulting in structural changes or lesions.

A diagnostic computer program must not only be able to diagnose diseases but also normality or health.

CONCATENATED EVENTS: ETIOLOGY, PATHOGENESIS, PATHOLOGY, PATHOPHYSIOLOGY, SYMPTOM, CLINICAL DATA, SYNDROME, COMPLICATION, CLINICAL PRESENTATION, CLINICAL ENTITY

Scientists believe in the principle of causality. Every cause has a corresponding effect; conversely, every effect presupposes a cause (except for the big bang for which we yet do not have a scientific explanation.)

Accordingly, every disease must have a cause. For many diseases, the causes are known; for others, they remain unknown. Even in the latter situation, we accept that a cause nevertheless must exist and we would propose theories regarding this cause. The discipline that studies the causes of diseases is **etiology**; if a diagnosis pinpoints a cause, we have an etiologic diagnosis—the diagnostic ideal. Determination of the cause is of great importance as it offers a possibility of a direct confrontation; elimination of the cause cures the patient, provided no irreversible anatomical changes have occurred. Sometimes, the term etiology is used as a synonym for cause of a specific disease.

From the moment a cause affects a healthy person and overcomes his defense mechanisms, a series of concatenated events occurs. Let's take the example of tuberculosis. The cause (*Mycobacterium tuberculosis*) produces toxins that alter the normal structure of the body and thereby produce lesions. The discipline that studies lesions is **pathology**; the mechanisms by which the cause produces lesions is

pathogenesis. Lesions result from changes in anatomical structure and physicochemical composition. They can be macroscopic, microscopic, or submicroscopic, and often are characteristic of the cause; however this does not always happen, as diverse causes can produce similar lesions. Lesions, in turn, modify normal function. *Physiology* is the discipline of normal function; **pathophysiology** is the study of the mechanisms by which a lesion causes abnormal function. Abnormal functioning is evidenced by several types of clues:

- **Symptoms**, in the strict medical sense, are subjective clues (*e.g.*, pain, nausea, vertigo) that the patient experiences. These clues are revealed by the patient during history taking.

- **Signs** are objective clues (*e.g.*, jaundice, swelling, wheezing) that a clinician detects during steps of the physical examination: inspection (observing the patient); palpation (feeling the shape, temperature, consistency, tenderness, of organs); percussion (tapping and listening to the elicited sound); auscultation (listening to sounds produced by organs); and other maneuvers. A patient may or may not be aware of his signs.

- **Results of tests, studies, or procedures** are clues obtained through laboratory tests, electrocardiograms, X-ray images, computed tomograms, sonograms, endoscopies, and other techniques.

Various synonyms (data, features, manifestations, traits, attributes, findings) are given to these clues that encompass symptoms, signs, and results of tests, studies, and procedures. We employ the term **clinical datum (pl. DATA)** to refer to any of these clues. Clinical data are indirect manifestations of the cause of a disease. All such clinical data are the result of the mentioned chain of events:

$$\text{CAUSE} \xrightarrow{\text{Pathogenesis}} \text{LESION} \xrightarrow{\text{Pathophysiology}} \text{CLINICAL DATA}$$

The described concatenation of events is perhaps too simplistic, because a single cause can provoke diverse and multiple lesions; each lesion can give rise to several pathophysiologic mechanisms, each yielding characteristic clinical data. This chain of events, although shown as a single straight path, actually is better represented as a tree (Fig. 1) with its trunk (cause), branches (pathogenesis and pathophysiology), and leaves (clinical data.) If additional links between these elements exist (dashed

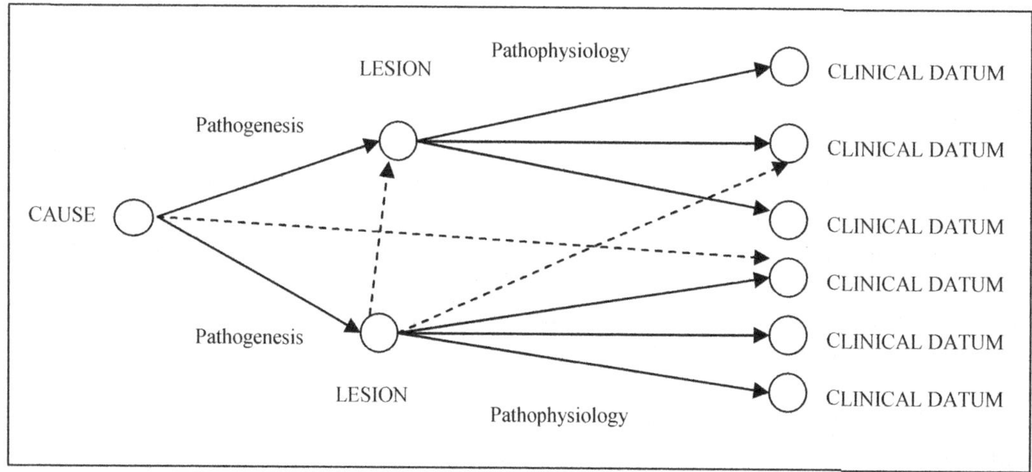

FIGURE 1. Chain of clinical events represented with a tree (solid arrows). Addition of dashed arrows creates an entangled network.

arrows in Fig. 1), the tree becomes an entangled network (*e.g.*, INTERNIST/CADUCEUS program by Myers, Pople, and Miller [13] [14].) Some authors (*e.g.*, Dana Ludwig's INFERNET program [15]) assign the probability with which the event occurs to each corresponding branch, node, and leaf.

In reality, lesion and clinical datum, same as pathogenic and pathophysiologic mechanisms may not always be clearly distinguishable. An apparent lesion itself becomes a clinical datum (*e.g.*, skin lesions of zoster or shingles.) Sometimes a cause directly provokes a clinical datum, without an apparent lesion (*e.g.*, a pyrogen that causes a fever.)

Causal or hierarchical trees or networks such as that described in Fig. 1 might be useful for didactic purposes because they help to organize knowledge. However, they are unsuitable for a comprehensive computer diagnosis program because they are complicated to implement and update, especially when combined with probabilities; furthermore, many pathogenic and pathophysiologic branches are unknown.

Clinical data tend to cluster into characteristic patterns called **syndromes** ("running together".) The clinical data that a syndrome comprises typically result from pathophysiologic mechanisms that originate in a common lesion. From the clinical data, tracing back these mechanisms leads to the diagnosis of the lesion.

A specific disease can produce more than one syndrome. For example, pancreatic cancer can manifest a bile duct obstruction syndrome (jaundice, increased serum bilirubin, choluria, pale stools), an anemic syndrome (paleness, low red blood cell count, fatigue), and a wasting syndrome (weight loss, emaciation, weakness.)

Concurrent diseases are those that simultaneously afflict a single patient. We call them **unrelated concurrent diseases** when the concurrence is random and one disease is completely independent from the other; **related concurrent diseases**, when dependence exists.

Complication is a secondary disease or medical condition that is a consequence of a primary disease. Typically, a lesion of the primary disease enables the action of a secondary cause producing the complication. Example 1: an ingrown nail (primary cause) that provokes a wound (primary lesion), which allows the entry of bacteria (secondary cause) provoking infection (secondary disease.) Example 2: primary peptic ulcer disease that causes a loss of stomach wall substance (primary lesion.) Should this lesion deepen and perforate the wall, the stomach contents would spill into the peritoneum and cause peritonitis (secondary disease, complication of the ulcer) with its own lesion (peritoneal inflammation) and clinical data (pain, guarding, rebound tenderness, etc.) Sometimes, doubt arises as to whether a manifestation should be considered either a syndrome or a complication of the primary disease, because no rigid difference exists between the two concepts. For example, some consider bleeding to be a clinical datum of peptic ulcer disease; others consider it a complication. Perhaps a manifestation of a disease should be considered a complication if uncommon, unexpected, unusually intense, or related to a lesion of the primary disease (*e.g.*, blood vessel wall erosion) rather than to its cause (stress, non-steroidal anti-inflammatory drugs [NSAID].)

A specific disease may present with diverse clinical pictures involving combinations of clinical data, syndromes, or complications. The intensity of the cause, the localization of the lesions produced, the time elapsed since the onset of the disease, and the patient's reaction, are responsible for such diverse clinical pictures. This diversity is referred to by several terms such as clinical presentation, clinical form, stage, or degree. I was unable to find formal definitions or clear-cut differences between these terms, some of which overlap. Here is how we use these terms in this publication:

Clinical form: one of the diverse constellations of clinical data manifested, resulting from a single cause or type of lesion. An *acute* form, displays symptoms that appear suddenly and briefly evolve toward a cure, chronicity, or death (*e.g.*, viral hepatitis.) A *chronic* form has a protracted course (*e.g.*, rheumatoid arthritis.) Some forms depend on *lesion localization* (*e.g.*, pulmonary, intestinal, renal, or genital tuberculosis.) Other forms depend on *lesion characteristics* (*e.g.*, fibrotic, caseous, miliary, or cavitary tuberculosis.)

Stage refers to the change of clinical data a disease presents over time. An example is syphilis that progresses through several stages, each with totally different syndromes that appear as if they pertain to unrelated diseases.

Degree refers to severity and often is related to duration and progression (stage) of the disease. Examples are congestive heart failure degrees I, II, III, and IV.

No clear-cut distinction exists among the concepts of syndrome, disease, and complication. Example 1: hyperthyroidism can be considered a disease with diverse causes, such as Graves' disease, toxic adenoma, TSH-secreting pituitary adenoma. These causes also can be considered diseases *per se*, in which case hyperthyroidism becomes a syndrome. Example 2: atrial fibrillation is a cardiac arrhythmia that can be considered either a disease (when no cause is found), a syndrome (of hyperthyroidism or myocardial ischemia), or a complication (of myocardial infarction). To refer to any of these elements we need a generic term, called clinical entity.

Complex clinical presentation: we reserve this term for cases where two or more final diagnoses are needed to account for all manifested clinical data. For example, coronary artery disease, acute myocardial infarction, congestive heart failure, shock, *and* thromboembolism in a single patient.

Clinical entity: a generic term for any element of a *complex clinical presentation*, such as a cause, lesion, syndrome, complication, disease, clinical form, stage, or degree.

The previous chain of events can now be expanded, tracking the provoking cause of a disease through a succession of causal relations to its final clinical presentation:

<pre>
            Pathogenesis   Pathophysiology
CAUSE ──────────────▶ LESION ──────────────────▶ CLINICAL DATA ──▶ SYNDROMES ──▶ CLINICAL PRESENTATION
</pre>

DISEASE MODEL

A **disease model** (Table 1), as defined in this study, is an abstract concept that comprises all clinical data that can be manifested by all patients with a specific disease. A single patient typically never manifests all clinical data that the disease potentially can provoke. Integration of a specific disease model with all of its possible manifestations requires statistical study of a large patient population. *Each clinical form, stage, and degree of disease has its own disease model.* Because health, death, and iatrogenic diseases are diagnoses that must be established clinically, the corresponding disease models must also be created.

Clinical data pertinent to a disease model can be collected either retrospectively or prospectively. Retrospectively, by reviewing medical records of past cases, journal articles, medical texts, etc. Prospectively, by accumulating clinical data from new cases; over time, the clinical data set will grow by apposition. This is related to the concept of "learning computers," where the computer gradually "learns" the disease, as the model progressively is refined.

DISEASE MODEL FOR ACUTE APPENDICITIS				
Symptoms	**S**	**PP value**	**Cost**	**Masked by**
Anorexia	0.93	0.20	none	
Pain in right lower abdomen	0.95	0.30	none	‡ (analgesics, antibiotics)
Vomiting	0.66	0.16	none	‡ (antiemetics)
Nausea	0.64	0.15	none	
Fever/chills	0.29	0.07	none	‡ (antipyretics, antibiotics)
Constipation	0.70	0.02	none	
⋮	⋮	⋮	⋮	
Signs				
Rebound tenderness	0.86	0.18	none	‡ (analgesics, antibiotics)
Fever (>37.5 C)	0.36	0.08	none	‡ (antitermics, antibiotics)
⋮	⋮	⋮	⋮	
Laboratory				
Increased white blood cell count	0.96	0.21	small	
Albumin in urine	0.19	0.04	small	
⋮	⋮	⋮	⋮	
Abdominal ultrasound				
Swollen appendix or abscess	0.60	0.95	intermediate	
⋮	⋮	⋮	⋮	
Laparotomy finding	1.00	1.00	great	

TABLE 1. Example of disease model; S, sensitivity (page 24); PP value, positive predictive value (page 25); cost of obtaining the clinical datum (page 29); ‡, interaction identifier (page 88.) The numeric values for S and PP value in the above examples were not obtained from actual statistics or calculations.

In addition to its primary diagnostic purpose to enable sorting out all diseases that can explain a given clinical datum, disease models also can provide the reciprocal information, listing all the clinical data that a given disease potentially can manifest. Disease models will be useful for study or research, if links to related medical information such as etiology, pathogenesis, pathology, pathophysiology, complications, prognosis, and treatment are created. All disease models are stored in the knowledge base.

Disease model may be confused with the corresponding **disease** that afflicts a patient. A disease model is a comprehensive clinical data list, while a disease is a malfunction of patient's organism.

DISEASE AND DIAGNOSIS

Disease and diagnosis frequently are ill defined, improperly applied with diverse meanings, or confused with each other.

Earlier, we defined **disease** as a condition in which some physicochemical parameter values are out of range and in which health qualities, such as well-being, harmony in all body functions, and the ability to establish and fulfill goals in life, are altered; in other words, *malfunction of the organism*. It typically leads to structural changes or lesions. This is a biological definition.

Diseases are named according to either a cause (giardiasis), a lesion (tuberculosis), an author who described it (Parkinson), a patient in whom it was observed (Pickwick), or a related occupation (farmer's lung.)

To a clinician, disease either refers to a specific disease that afflicts a patient or to the corresponding disease model.

Diagnosis also can be variously interpreted. It is defined as the identification of an abnormal condition that afflicts a specific patient, based on manifested clinical data or lesions. The chain of events going from the cause of a disease to the resulting clinical data or clinical presentation is shown on page 12. Diagnosis denotes the *physician's mental process* that, starting with clinical presentation, progresses toward the cause of the disease, reversing the direction of the chain of events described above:

CLINICAL PRESENTATION ⟶ SYNDROMES ⟶ CLINICAL DATA $\xrightarrow{\text{Pathophysiology}}$ LESION $\xrightarrow{\text{Pathogenesis}}$ CAUSE

Alternatively, diagnosis may refer only to the end result of the diagnostic process: if the clinician is able to retrogradely traverse the chain of events, from the clinical presentation or the clinical data to the cause, he obtains an *etiologic diagnosis*. This is optimal, because it typically enables elimination of the cause and accomplishes a cure. If he only attains the lesion level, he obtains a *pathologic or anatomic diagnosis* that may still enable satisfactory treatment. If he is unable to proceed beyond the clinical data level, he obtains a *symptomatic diagnosis*, which only enables a less desirable palliative or empirical treatment (*e.g.*, fever or pain relief.)

The concepts of disease and diagnosis, as defined by us, are graphically represented in Fig. 2, on next page. When a *final diagnosis* agrees with a *disease* that afflicts a patient, the diagnostic process is correct; otherwise, a misdiagnosis occurred. This figure also shows how *syndromes* relate to *lesions*.

Associations occurring in the physician's mind during the diagnostic process are evoked by his memory, recalling knowledge acquired during his study of medicine and experience with actual cases of diseased patients.

Diagnosis can be considered in yet another way. Any diagnostic algorithm conceived is likely to be based on disease models stored in the computer knowledge base or in the physician's memory, including the name of the disease with the cause, pathogenesis, lesions, pathophysiology, clinical data, syndromes, clinical presentations, and complications. Then, all available information from a specific patient is collected and compared with all disease models. When a successful match between the patient's clinical data and those included in a disease model is achieved, the patient's disease has been diagnosed. This interpretation is related to pattern recognition and perhaps is one way the human mind solves the diagnostic problem; artificial intelligence emulates this process with computers.

Two major obstacles complicate matching of patient clinical data and disease model clinical data:

1. A disease typically manifests not all of the clinical data included in its disease model. The quantity and quality of manifested clinical data depend in part on patient idiosyncrasy, the severity of the cause, and the site, number, and magnitude of the lesions. This makes diagnosis difficult. Incomplete expression of a disease can be compared to a criminal who leaves behind only a fragment of a fingerprint or a partial sequence of DNA. Additional investigated clues, when integrated with primary ones, provide a broader picture that may enable identification of the culprit. Similarly, inapparent additional clinical data can be investigated, although at an increased cost, to attain the diagnosis of the disease that afflicts the patient.

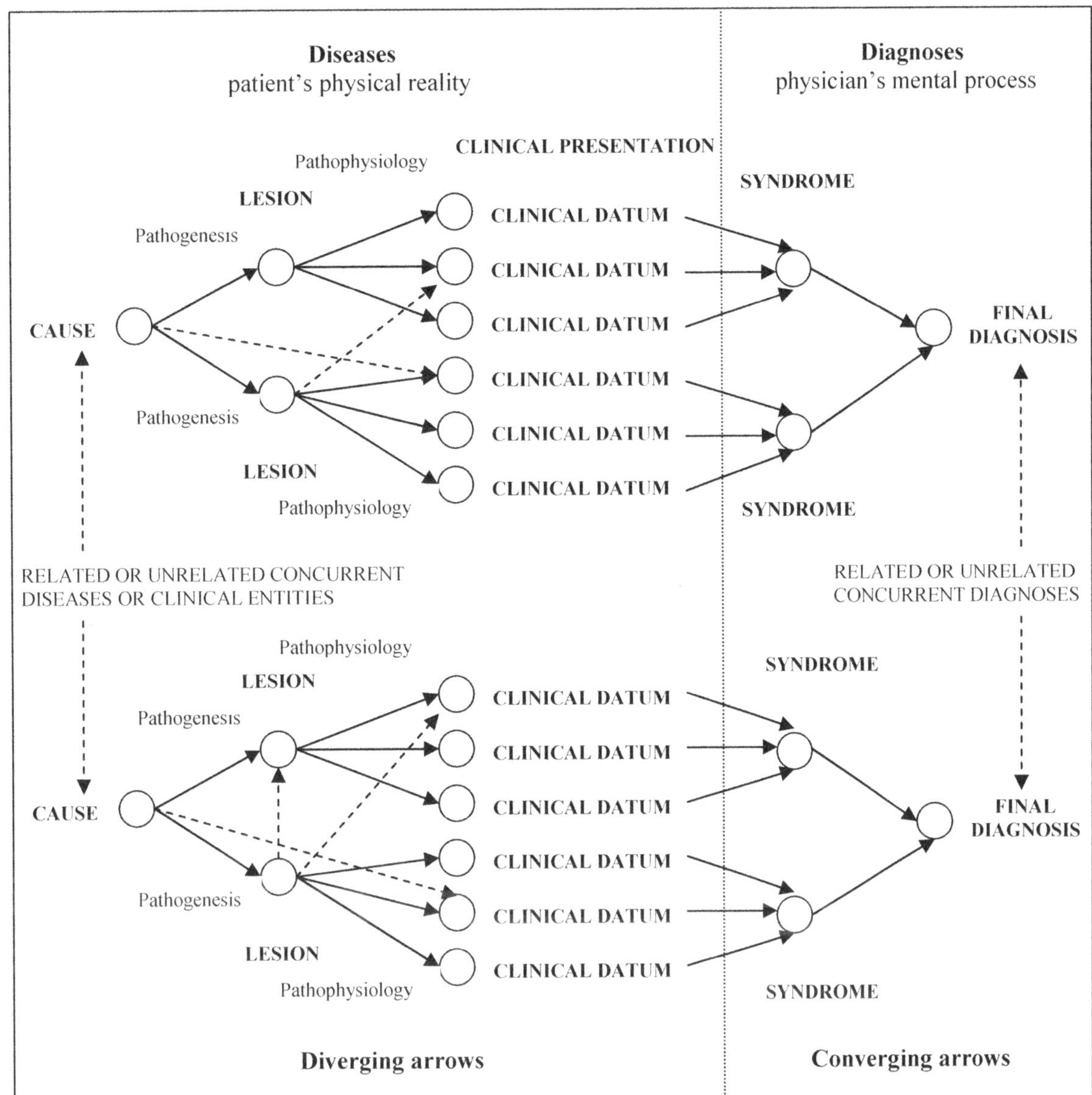

FIGURE 2. Tree (solid arrows) or network (solid and dashed arrows) representing the chain of clinical events occurring in a patient during a disease (left side of figure) and the associations occurring in the mind of a physician during a diagnostic process (right side of the figure).

2. No one-to-one correspondence exists between patient clinical data and disease model clinical data, because the former often are not exclusive for a single disease. Unfortunately, several diseases may manifest similar clinical data (*e.g.*, obstruction of the common bile duct by a gallstone may cause jaundice similar to that caused by a tumor; intestinal bleeding may be caused by cancer, trauma, or an ulcer.) Such sharing of clinical data by diverse diseases creates confusion, making selection of the correct diagnosis from the list of *competing diagnoses* difficult for the physician and computer alike. This problem is compounded when the patient is afflicted by more than one disease (*concurrent diseases*.) We will deal with these problems later.

Do not confuse the terms disease and diagnosis. Sometimes, we wrongly apply these terms interchangeably: for example pneumonia disease for pneumonia diagnosis and vice versa. A disease is a *change in the patient's body*, whereas a diagnosis is a *physician's mental construct* (Fig. 2.) Contradicting diseases (*e.g.*, hyperthyroidism and hypothyroidism) cannot coexist in a given patient, but these two diagnoses could conceivably exist in the same differential diagnosis list, but with different probabilities, because both diseases may share certain symptoms (*e.g.*, pretibial edema.) This confusion leads some computer program researchers to wrongly eliminate one of these apparently contradicting diagnoses from the differential diagnosis list.

In summary, when taken out of context, the distinction between disease and diagnosis may be uncertain. Does disease refer to a specific patient's problem or to its corresponding disease model? Does diagnosis refer to the mental process that leads to the identification of a disease or to the final suspicion of a cause, lesion, or syndrome? These meanings must be discriminated by the physician's mind and by a computer algorithm.

In the context of our research, *diagnosis* means probability of disease. This definition refers properly to *potential diagnosis*; whereas the dictionary definition—the identification of an abnormal condition that afflicts a specific patient, based on manifested clinical data—is what we call a *final diagnosis*. Unless otherwise qualified, *diagnosis* will denote *potential diagnosis*.

Disease prevalence is the fraction of a population afflicted by a specific disease at a specific time. It also can be interpreted as the likelihood of a person belonging to that population to be afflicted by that disease.

MEDICAL EXAMINATION

Medical examination is the process by which initial clinical data are collected. Physicians traditionally do this in a systematic fashion to preclude missing important information. A medical record typically comprises the following sections:

General information

Name, date of birth, sex, ethnicity, street address, date of examination, record number, etc.

Medical history

Present illness: first, the patient is asked to enumerate and describe his current symptoms; then, appropriate questions are asked to target specific diagnoses. These questions must be easily understandable by the patient; the physician translates the answers into technical terminology and documents them in the medical record. Positive symptoms (affirmed by the patient) and negative symptoms (denied by the patient) are noted.

As an example, I will list the symptoms related to specific organs or systems that I routinely ask my patients; this procedure is used by most physicians, but other valid approaches also exist. These questions should cover important symptoms and not be unduly abbreviated, as in managed care style. If diagnostic suspicions arise, then appropriately detailed and focused questions can be asked.

My list includes: headache, dizziness, earache and hearing problems, vision problems, nasal congestion, sinus pain, sore throat; cough, sputum production, shortness of breath, chest pain, palpitation; nausea and vomiting, abdominal pain, bowel movements, black stools; bleeding from any source, swollen legs or puffy eyelids, frequency or other difficulty with urination; musculoskeletal pain, any swelling or deformity, appetite, excessive thirst and urination, weight change, mental status or mood change, socioeconomic status, and education. For women, I also ask about menarche, menstrual abnormalities, menopause, and vaginal itching or discharge. For men, I also ask about urethral discharge, sexual function and sexual orientation (if pertinent.)

Many physicians also document normal observations and important absent symptoms, under the heading *review of systems* or *review of symptoms.*

Some symptoms may have diverse non-exclusive qualities. For example, pain can be constrictive, burning, throbbing, stabbing, or excruciating. Each of these qualities may have diagnostic implications. This creates a computational dilemma: either we consider each quality as a distinct clinical datum characteristic of a specific disease, or categorically ignore symptom quality because it is subjective (varies according to patient perception.) However, some qualities are so characteristic that they cannot be ignored; for example brief chest pain favors a diagnosis of angina pectoris, whereas sustained chest pain suggests myocardial infarction.

Past history: next, an inquiry should be made into the patient's prior medical problems. Such information might reveal that the present illness represents a stage, a complication, or a sequel of a previous problem.

Family history: may provide clues concerning genetic or developmental factors that predispose the present illness.

Social history: alerts to toxic or environmental causes of diseases such as smoking, alcoholism, drugs, stress, job or profession, habits and diet that may relate to the present illness.

History taking can be challenging. On the part of physician, it requires skill, experience, patience, time, compassion, understanding of human nature, and often a kind of Buddhist benevolence. A computer cannot yet provide these qualities. On the part of the patient, most are intelligent and cultured, which makes the history taking easy and pleasant. Others answer each medical question with an exuberant list of complaints, embellished with social life details. Neurotic patients tend to answer affirmatively every question regarding symptoms. Still other patients, on the contrary, would hide or ignore their symptoms that can be retrieved only with great insistence. Malingerers and patients with severe mental problems can be especially difficult.

Not all history information needs to be entered in the computer. A primary purpose for asking so many questions is to remind the patient about relevant clinical data that he forgot or considered unimportant.

Physical examination

The physical examination that follows also must be methodical. The procedure is well established; as with history taking, it roughly follows a regional order from head to toe, and often is organ or system oriented. The methods used to examine a patient (page 10) are inspection, palpation, percussion, auscultation, and specific maneuvers. The most important aspects of the examination are:

Vital signs: pulse, blood pressure, respiration, and temperature.

General signs: nutrition, weight and stature, development, mental status.

Head: paranasal sinus tenderness, nostrils, eyelids, conjunctivae and eyes, gross vision, pupils and pupillary reflexes, funduscopy, gross hearing, otoscopy, mouth including hygiene and dental status, throat, and tonsils.

Neck: suppleness, range of motion, lymph node swelling and tenderness, masses, salivary glands, vein distension, trachea, thyroid gland, arterial pulses and bruits.

Chest: lungs, heart, mediastinum, diaphragm; axilla and supraclavicular regions: lymph node swelling; breasts.

Abdomen: liver, spleen, kidneys, intestine, masses, tension, tenderness, rebound tenderness, ascites, hernias, and rectal examination, if indicated (digital rectal examination and anoscopy).

Extremities: pulses, veins, swelling, signs of deep venous thrombosis, trophism.

Gross neurologic exam: strength, reflexes, sensation, coordination, cranial nerves, Babinski and Romberg signs.

Osteoarticular and *muscular systems*: deformities, inflammation, tenderness.

Lymphatic system: lymph node enlargement, tenderness, consistency, shape, mobility, overlying skin status.

Skin: trophism, color, temperature, tenderness, swelling, collateral circulation, specific lesions.

Genitalia (men): testicles, rectal palpation for prostate (age 50 and over); (women): pelvic exam and Papanicolaou smear.

The physical examination must be accomplished sensitively, with respect and decorum. As with the history, this information is documented, describing positive signs and mentioning important negative signs.

Finally, a **diagnostic assessment** and a **plan** for diagnostic studies and initial treatment, complete the medical record. This traditional method of clinical data collection is still accomplished by conscientious physicians who are not pressed by time limitations or other restrictions. Perhaps the computer, via heuristic shortcuts, will enable a more efficient method that will be straightforwardly oriented towards the diagnostic goal. Many efforts have been undertaken to create computerized storage of medical records, written with a unified terminology, easily and universally retrievable by all authorized parties; but success and acceptability in this field is at present only partial.

An important point to keep in mind is that even if we have a high probability and convincing final diagnosis, a patient might have yet another occult disease in addition to the apparent one. For this reason, the medical history and the physical examination must always be as complete as possible. From the first to the last day of my 50 years of medical practice, I was always concerned that I might miss such occult diseases. With my usual compulsion I did this complete physical examination with **all** my patients. A friend of my family jokingly remarked that, if one consult Dr. Feder for a sore throat, he would remove your underwear. This habit paid good dividends because, in many cases, it enabled me to unveil diseases that were overlooked by colleagues. This is neither boastfulness nor criticism, but reality; fortunately, I did not have to depend much on managed care with its many restrictions. This translates to a need to not only accomplish a diagnostic search for a patient's specific disease, but also a comprehensive study, following specific guidelines outlined in the next section. Ideally, both activities should be done at the same appointment.

HEALTH ASSESSMENT AND EARLY DETECTION OF DISEASE

A healthy patient has no complaints and no abnormal clinical data. However, patients sometimes ignore or underestimate their symptoms, or even hide them for social or legal reasons. Also, many diseases are occult, at least in their early stages. Health diagnosis mandates a comprehensive history and physical examination identical to that described for disease diagnosis, only that we have no initial clues for possible disease. If some clinical datum is unveiled during the history or physical examination, even though it might seem irrelevant or unimportant (*e.g.*, a mild tension headache), we are obliged to enter it in the computer, so that the diagnostic program can evaluate it. If the history and physical examination are so far completely normal, the patient still could have an occult or incipient disease, such as diabetes, lipid abnormalities, or cancer, which often are asymptomatic in their early stages. Early detection of these occult diseases offers a better chance for cure. Consequently, despite a normal history and physical examination, health assessment and early detection of disease mandate additional clinical studies to improve diagnostic accuracy.

Health diagnosis presents the same problem as diagnosing overt disease, namely how many and what kind of tests and procedures would provide reasonable confidence that the patient indeed is healthy and all possible occult diseases have been ruled out. No ideal solution exists to this problem, because medicine is an inexact science. Even were a patient subjected to all currently available tests and diagnostic procedures—a practical impossibility—a disease still could be missed. When one should stop considering further diagnostic efforts is unclear. For an apparently normal person, one cannot request biopsies of all his organs, a laparoscopy, or other invasive and costly procedures. The limit of such efforts depends on the seriousness of the medical situation, patient age and sex, risk factors, financial status, willingness to submit to recommend procedures, insurance company approval, involved liability, and many other factors. This issue is beyond the scope of this essay.

My routine work-up for otherwise uncomplicated cases comprises: a comprehensive medical history and physical examination, blood analysis, including CBC, ESR, glucose, BUN, creatinine, electrolytes with calcium, total serum protein, albumin, liver panel with enzymes, lipid panel, iron, transferrin, TIBC, uric acid, TSH, and urinalysis. In men, after age 50, I recommend an electrocardiogram, PSA, and, when indicated, chest X-rays and fecal occult blood. For women, mammograms and pelvic examination including a Pap smear. I recommend regular breast self-examinations. For other procedures directed at early detection of disease such as colonoscopy, readers should consult specialty guidelines. Routine medical examinations primarily focus on usually chronic occult diseases, which if left untreated will result in serious complications or a dismal prognosis, that justify additional studies based on their costs and benefits. As mentioned, examples of diseases that may be occult are lipid abnormalities, diabetes, and cancer.

Malingering and hypochondriasis are diagnoses that a computer algorithm should be able to detect. It is suspected whenever clinical data do not converge to a single diagnosis or combination of diagnoses. This situation mandates a comprehensive work-up, including a comprehensive medical examination, laboratory tests, or other diagnostic procedures, which would be expected to be within normal limits.

PRINCIPLES OF OUR DIAGNOSTIC COMPUTER PROGRAM

To create our diagnostic algorithm, we departed from the principles that it must be simple—avoiding complicated mathematical formulas—able to be understood by physicians and computer scientists alike, and easy to update. To comply with these principles, we concluded that it must emulate, as close as possible, the natural medical reasoning. We also comprehended the need of a firm ground on which to buildup this algorithm, and considered sensitivity (S)—frequency with which a specific disease manifests a specific clinical datum—a reliable ground. Sensitivity is obtainable through statistics, which depends on the number of cases analyzed and correct tabulation of findings. Despite inaccuracy of statistical calculations, we believe that no better ground than sensitivity exists to our purpose.

CATEGORICAL AND PROBABILISTIC REASONING IN MEDICAL DIAGNOSIS

Whether a computer program should be more categorical (deterministic) or more probabilistic (mathematical) has been repeatedly discussed in the medical diagnosis literature [16]. We are convinced that a diagnostic algorithm must be predominantly categorical. I will insist in later sections that mathematical formulas like the Bayes theorem do not work well for the intended purpose. Physicians in general have great curiosity; they want to know the why, what, where, and when of a diagnosis. They do not trust black boxes with esoteric formulas that yield a diagnosis; they want to know what is inside the box. They want to know details such as clinical presentation, syndromes, pathophysiology, lesion, pathogenesis, and cause. In addition to diagnosing, an algorithm that provides these details can be useful for teaching and research.

Another problem is that probabilities are based on statistics, and medical statistics often are inaccurate and difficult to obtain. Prevalence of a disease—the frequency with which a disease exists among a population—is determined statistically; but many cases are not reported. Sensitivity of a clinical datum for a specific disease—fraction of patients with the disease who manifest the clinical datum—require the study of a quite large population of patients. Perlroth and Weiland, in their book FIFTY DISEASES: FIFTY DIAGNOSES [17] retrospectively reviewed approximately 1,000 patient records for each of 50 diseases (1,000 X 50 = 50,000 records) and determined the sensitivity of each clinical datum. To accomplish the same task for the approximately 4,000 currently known diseases would require reviewing 1,000 X 4,000 = 4,000,000 patient records. This is why no consensus exists among authors regarding the magnitude of diverse sensitivities, which is often based on anecdotal experience. However, accurate sensitivity data are important for many computer diagnostic programs, and ours is no exception. Determination of the sensitivities of all clinical data for all diseases must be accomplished by a medical team. Essential rule:

A diagnostic algorithm must essentially be based on categorical reasoning, with the fewest possible mathematical calculations, and provide cross-references to additional information such as etiology, pathogenesis, pathology, pathophysiology, syndromes, etc.

In conclusion, after my best efforts to analyze the complex mental mechanisms of diagnosing—partially conscious and partially unconscious with obscure relations to intuition—I came up with two principal models. The first, which could be called a causal diagnostic process, is based on the described chain of events:

CAUSE —(Pathogenesis)→ LESION —(Pathophysiology)→ CLINICAL DATA → SYNDROMES → CLINICAL PRESENTATION

If we knew, for all diseases, all details of this cascade of events, then we could achieve a diagnosis by traversing backwards the chain of events from the clinical presentation to the cause, as mentioned earlier. Unfortunately, medicine is an incomplete science, and many links in this chain of events are as yet unknown, especially in complex clinical situations. As difficult as it is to unveil many of these pathogenic and pathophysiologic links, to determine the probabilities with which they occur is even more complicated. Such incomplete knowledge renders unrealistic the implementation of the entire medicine with this diagnostic model, represented by trees, networks, and probabilities associated with their branches, nodes, and leaves. At best, it may be applicable to simple syndromes and to limited specialized areas of internal medicine [18] [19] [20], but not to complex clinical presentations.

The second model—pattern-matching diagnostic process—compares a specific patient's clinical data with the clinical data of all disease models. The best match is the final diagnosis. This model, despite its inherent difficulties—partial manifestation of patient clinical data and a lack of univocal (one-to-one) match of patient clinical data with disease model clinical data (page 14)—would appear to be a practical approach to computer emulation of the human diagnostic process.

A mathematical model that attempts to represent with esoteric formulas, matrices, or vectors the many complex diagnostic situations and nuances is divorced from clinical reality.

HEURISTIC VERSUS EXHAUSTIVE SEARCH FOR MEDICAL INFORMATION

Heuristics consider problem-solving methods, based on experience, rules of thumb, insight, or intuition, for simplifying and shortening a computer process, as opposed to an algorithm of **exhaustive** searching, collecting, and processing of information.

Diagnostic reasoning—whether by physicians or computers—is affected by two opposing forces. On one hand, the more clinical data gathered and potential diagnoses processed, the less likely we are to miss an occult disease that might threaten life or expose health care providers to liability. On the other hand, exhaustive collection of medical information is prohibitive because of the incurred cost—price, discomfort, and risk—and processing burden.

Our diagnostic algorithm is based on the emulation of human medical reasoning; accordingly, it uses many heuristic methods as seen in following sections.

DISREGARD QUALITIES OF CLINICAL DATA

Clinical data, especially subjective symptoms, typically have diverse non-exclusive qualities. For example, chest pain of angina pectoris typically is retrosternal, radiating to the neck, jaw, and upper extremities; is oppressive, lasting only a few minutes; is exertion related and relieved by nitroglycerine. Some authors confer values to these pain qualities, their chronology, and their evolution. This is correct, when such qualities, powerfully suggest a diagnosis. Nevertheless, our algorithm purposely *does not consider such clinical data qualities*; we believe that computation of clinical datum qualities is not critical for calculation of probability of a diagnosis. Reasons are: clinical data qualities and chronology are subjective and widely variable; chest pain of angina pectoris sometimes is mild, referred to the upper abdomen, not radiating, is burning, or even absent in patients with diabetes. Accordingly, these qualities may not be reliable. Anxious or hypochondriac patients can imagine such qualities. To confirm angina pectoris, more reliable tests, such as stress ECG and sometimes angiogram are needed, which provide clinical data with greater supporting value that anyway will supersede the oppressive quality of chest pain that has a lesser supporting value. Disregarding these unreliable qualities simplifies the diagnostic process without losing accuracy. It would be difficult, if not impossible, to determine the sensitivity (see page 21), necessary to calculate the supporting positive predictive value (page 25), of each diverse quality that thousand of known clinical data and diseases can manifest. In the especial case where the quality of a clinical datum is essential, such as the mentioned case of prolonged retrosternal pain for myocardial infarction, this quality can be included as a separate clinical datum in the corresponding disease model. Essential rule:

Disregard clinical data qualities in computer diagnosis programs.

DISREGARD DISEASE PREVALENCE

Prevalence of a disease is the number of existing cases in a given population at a specific time. Prevalence statistics are of epidemiological importance. However, it may be harmful to include prevalence values when calculating the probability of a patient having a rare disease. This happens because the small prevalence value for such a rare disease could considerably reduce the probability of the corresponding diagnosis, causing it to be improperly ruled out. If a patient has a disease afflicting only one in a million persons, the probability of that diagnosis would be very small, but for him it represents one hundred percent. A perfect program should diagnose every possible disease, including those that are rare. After all, we do not need a computer to diagnose a common cold during an epidemic. Furthermore, accurate epidemiological information is difficult to obtain because many disease cases remain unreported. Accordingly, our diagnostic algorithm purposely does *not* take prevalence into account; this is equivalent to assuming that all diseases occur with the same probability. Essential rule:

Disregard prevalence or prior probability of diseases in computer diagnosis programs.

SYNONYMS OF CLINICAL DATA

Clinical data terms must be recognized and accepted by the algorithm. A given clinical datum can be referred to by different synonyms (*e.g.*, shortness of breath, dyspnea, or respiratory distress.) Standard terms for clinical data, for example Medical Subject Headings (MeSH) or Systematized Nomenclature of Medicine (SNOMED) are preferred, but if a synonym is used, the algorithm must be able to translate it into an acceptable standard term. When this happens, the user is notified; if no match is found, he is prompted to try another synonym. This synonym problem is addressed in the RECONSIDER program (Blois, *et al* [25]). Essential rule:

For clinical data, use standard terms or synonyms that are recognized by the algorithm.

INDICES AND IDENTIFIERS OF CLINICAL DATA

In our knowledge base, three **indices** are associated with each clinical datum: *sensitivity, positive predictive value*, and *cost*; two **identifiers** are associated with selected clinical data: *risk* and *interaction identifiers*.

Indices

1. *Sensitivity* (S)

Sensitivity is defined as the conditional probability P of a clinical datum C, given a disease D:

$$S = P\,(C|D) \tag{1}$$

Where: S = sensitivity of clinical datum C for disease D

A practical way to calculate S of a specific clinical datum for a given disease is to determine statistically the fraction of patients afflicted by this disease who manifest the clinical datum:

$$\text{Sensitivity (S)} = \frac{\text{Number of disease cases manifesting the clinical datum}}{\text{Total number of disease cases}} \tag{2}$$

Sensitivity can be expressed either as a decimal (*e.g.*, 0.30), or as a percentage (*e.g.*, 30%.)

A given clinical datum can be manifested by more than one disease. Accordingly, both the clinical datum and the disease that manifests it, determine the value of S. This value is stored in the knowledge base linked to the corresponding clinical datum and disease model.

If the numerator and denominator of equation 2 are equal, the sensitivity (S) of the datum will equal 1, which is unlikely, as it requires that all clinical cases so far reviewed manifested the clinical datum. Otherwise, the numerator will always be smaller than the denominator, S will be smaller than 1, and an additional clinical case will increase S if the clinical datum is present, or reduce it if the datum is absent. Accordingly, the computer recalculates the sensitivity of each clinical datum each time the knowledge base is updated with new cases. The greater the number of cases analyzed, the greater the accuracy of S. If a clinical datum never is manifested by a specific disease, its S equals 0 for this disease. When sufficient number of cases have been reviewed, the disease model will include all the clinical data this disease can potentially manifest, and the sensitivities will approach their true values.

Determination of S can be accomplished by (a) retrospectively incorporating information from past medical records and publications; (b) prospectively incorporating information from future medical records. The latter task would be an ongoing project; it would be facilitated by universal electronic storage and processing of medical records; (c) basing the sensitivities on the personal estimation of clinicians and specialists, but this is subjective and inaccurate. Retrospective, prospective, or estimative method is labor intensive and requires the cooperation of a medical team; the expected great benefits of such a medical resource are worth the effort.

To calculate S of a clinical datum, retrospectively or prospectively, one must trust the information source. If the physician who originally examines a patient overlooks or forgets to register a clinical datum, that datum would improperly be considered absent, and would render the calculation inaccurate.

To update the knowledge base, the computer program must:

- Add a new disease model, when a new disease is discovered.

- Add a new clinical datum to an existing disease model, when this datum is established with a novel test or procedure.

- Occasionally recalculate the sensitivity of clinical data when additional clinical cases are available.

As mentioned earlier (page 21), Perlroth and Weiland did an amazing job in their book "Fifty Diseases: Fifty Diagnoses", determining the frequency of each clinical datum for 50 diseases. These values were useful to test our diagnostic algorithm that is based essentially on clinical data sensitivities. When synonyms for a clinical datum are used (*e.g.*, dyspnea, shortness of breath, and respiratory distress) the physician and the computer algorithm must recognize that they refer to the same clinical datum; otherwise, each synonym would be assigned a different sensitivity, which is wrong. Another error sometimes encountered is assigning sensitivity to a syndrome (*e.g.*, congestive heart failure) instead to each of its component clinical data (*e.g.*, dyspnea, bibasal rales, hepatomegaly, edema.) The algorithm must diagnose the syndrome and calculate the corresponding probability of the diagnosis, based on the sensitivity of the component clinical data. Essential rule:

Do not assign sensitivity (S) to a syndrome, but only to its corresponding clinical data and let the algorithm calculate the probability (P) of such syndrome.

2. *Positive predictive value* (PP value)

Next, it was necessary to define an index that represents the strength with which each clinical datum present in the patient supports a specific diagnosis. S cannot be used directly because it only expresses how frequently a disease manifests a clinical datum, but not how often it occurs with other diseases. We consider that positive predictive value (PP value) best accomplishes this function. PP value is defined as the conditional probability P of a disease D, given a clinical datum present C:

$$PP \text{ value} = P\,(D|C) \tag{3}$$

Let's start with Bayes formula, which calculates conditional probabilities. Thomas Bayes (1702-1761), a theologian and a mathematician proposed his formula that was posthumously published in 1763. To my knowledge, Ledley and Lusted [21] [22] [23] first employed Bayes formula for the calculation of the probability of a specific diagnosis, given a clinical datum:

$$P\,(D_i|C) = \frac{P\,(D_i)\,P\,(C|D_i)}{P\,(D_1)\,P\,(C|D_1) + \ldots + P\,(D_i)\,P\,(C|D_i) + \ldots + P\,(D_n)\,P\,(C|D_n)} \tag{4}$$

Where: $P\,(D_i)$ = probability of disease D_i; also called *prior probability* because it is the probability of the disease *before* considering clinical datum C

$P\,(D_i|C)$ = probability of disease D_i, given specific clinical datum C; also called *posterior probability* of the disease because it is the result of the equation *after* considering clinical datum C

$D_1 \ldots D_n$ = all diseases that manifest clinical datum C, including D_i

$P\,(C|D)$ = probability of clinical datum C, given a disease D; it equals the sensitivity (S) of the clinical datum for this disease D: $P(C|D) = S$. This is valid for any disease $(D_1 \ldots D_n)$ that manifests clinical datum C

The probability of a clinical datum for a given disease equals the sensitivity of the clinical datum for this disease (equation 1.)

We explained earlier (page 23) the reasons why we purposely do not take into account prevalence of diseases, called prior probability of diseases in Bayesian context. This is equivalent to assuming that all diseases have the same prior probability [P (D)]; accordingly, we can simplify equation 4 by deleting the prior probability of all diseases [P (D$_1$)...P (D$_i$)...P (D$_n$)]. Then, if we replace P (D|C) with PP value (according to equation 3), and P (C|D) with S (according to equation 1), we obtain the following equation:

$$PP\ value_i \; = \; \frac{S_i}{S_1 + ... + S_i + ... + S_n} \tag{5}$$

Where: PP value$_i$ = positive predictive value of the clinical datum for the disease i under consideration

S$_i$ = sensitivity of the clinical datum for the disease i under consideration

S$_1$...S$_n$ = sensitivities of the *same clinical datum* for corresponding diseases*

* "Corresponding diseases" could either refer only to diseases that manifest the clinical datum, or alternatively to all known diseases. For either of these alternatives, the result will be identical, because S of a clinical datum for a disease that never manifests such datum is zero. Adding zeros to the value of the denominator established by S of the diseases that manifest the clinical datum will neither change the value of the denominator nor the result of the equation.

Equation 5 shows that S$_i$ (numerator of the right member) and PP value$_i$ are directly proportional.

This equation is convenient because it expresses PP value as a function of sensitivities (S), being S the cornerstone of our algorithm.

PP value = 1 when the clinical datum is manifested only by the disease under consideration (that is, when for all other diseases S = 0); conversely, PP value approaches 0 when the clinical datum is always manifested in all other diseases (that is, when for all other diseases S = 1), a theoretical situation. In remaining situations, PP value takes an intermediate value between 0 and 1.

PP value quantifies how characteristic or exclusive a clinical datum is for a specific disease or diagnosis. According to equation 5, the fewer the number of diseases that manifest a given clinical datum (number of S terms in the denominator) and the fewer this clinical datum is manifested by each of these diseases (the smaller each S value in the denominator), the greater the PP value of the clinical datum and the probability of the specific diagnosis or disease. For example, the presence of *Mycobacterium tuberculosis* in sputum is pathognomonic of pulmonary tuberculosis because no other disease manifests this clinical datum; accordingly PP value = 1. We believe that *PP value is the most accurate index of how strongly a clinical datum present supports a diagnosis or disease.*

Calculated PP values are linked to the corresponding clinical data in the disease models. Because PP values are based on statistically established sensitivities stored in the knowledge base, they do not depend on specific clinical cases, and therefore can be pre-calculated (before the diagnostic program is applied to actual clinical cases) saving computing real time. These values remain fixed unless new disease models are added to the knowledge base or revised statistics change the values of the sensitivities upon which PP values are based. Should such changes occur as a result of an occasional update, all PP values must be recalculated.

Definition of PP value based on equation 5 is rational, simple, accurate, practical, and novel.

As a consequence of Ledley and Lusted's efforts, Bayes formula has become extensively used in medical applications. However, when improperly applied in a diagnostic algorithm, as often is the case, it can cause significant inaccuracies.

Bayes formula is valid only when three conditions are fulfilled [13] [22] [23]:

1. Clinical data used for calculation of the conditional probability of a diagnosis must be **independent**: that is, a specific clinical datum should neither favor nor disfavor any other clinical datum of the same disease. In other words, the probability that one clinical datum is manifested by a specific disease, should not depend on the presence of another clinical datum. This is not true in actual clinical cases, where clinical data result from a chain of reactions that originate in a common cause or lesion and are necessarily related. These clinical data configure syndromes that by definition are associations of related clinical data (*e.g.*, jaundice, increased blood bilirubin, and dark urine.) The inaccuracy of Bayes formula for calculating the posterior probability of a diagnosis given clinical data that are *not independent* has been recognized by several researchers. Their excuse for using Bayes despite this realization is that they consider the introduced error not to substantially affect the final result [26]. Our criterion perhaps exaggerates in the opposite direction by considering that all clinical data manifested by a specific syndrome or disease are related and that independence of some clinical data would not significantly affect the final result. Ideally, our criterion should be applied only to related clinical data, and Bayes formula or other scoring system applied only to proven independent clinical data, but this relation or independence is often difficult to establish or is unknown. Essential rule:

Do not use Bayes formula to calculate the probability of a diagnosis.

2. The diseases must be **incompatible,** which means that clinical data justified by one disease cannot be justified by another disease. When concurrent diseases occur, some clinical data may be caused by more than one of them. Bayes formula is only capable to calculate probabilities of competing diagnosis, which are incompatible because only one can become a final diagnosis; consequently, it is unsuitable to handle concurrent diseases. When applied to concurrent diseases Bayes tries to explain all the manifested clinical data with a single diagnosis, considering all other diagnoses as competing; obviously, this yields an erroneous probability of such diagnosis. To solve the problems of independence and incompatibility, so-called Bayesian networks have been devised, but their application to diagnostic algorithms is excessively complicated and difficult to compute. We created the mini-max procedure (to be explained later), which identifies concurrent diagnoses despite manifesting shared clinical data, and calculates P of such diagnoses independently, circumventing the *incompatibility* condition of Bayes' formula.

3. The number of diseases (corresponding diagnoses) processed by the formula must be **exhaustive**: all known diseases must be included in the knowledge base, enabling inclusion in the denominator of all diagnoses that manifest the considered clinical datum. Should a disease be omitted, its disease model will not be created and the sensitivities of the corresponding clinical data will not be available and will miss from the denominator in equation 4 or 5. Consequently, the calculation of the PP value will be inaccurate; still worse, the diagnosis of the excluded disease will never be included in the differential diagnosis list. This is why computer programs based on Bayes formula but circumscribed to a restricted area of diseases—such as congenital cardiopathies or nephropathies—are inherently inaccurate. Essential rule:

To be accurate, a computer program must include and process *all* known diseases.

Equation 5 (page 26) that calculates PP values of clinical data derives from Bayes formula, when deleting the prior probabilities. This equation does not violate the aforementioned conditions because it includes in its denominator S of all known diseases capable of manifesting the clinical datum, complying with the *exhaustive* condition. These S refer to clinical data pertaining to unrelated disease models (as opposed to a specific patient) complying with the *independent* condition.

Bayesian concepts and equations typically are used by other diagnostic algorithms, which we do *not* endorse. The details discussed here refer to these alternate applications and are intended for educational purposes only; the reader may skip them without compromising his understanding of our algorithm.

Many authors use Bayes formula to calculate how each clinical datum changes the probability of a diagnosis. This probability, before considering any given clinical datum (*i.e.*, before applying Bayes formula), is called *prior probability* $[P(D_i)]$; it equals the prevalence of the disease (page 16) $[P(D) = $ prevalence of $D]$. Each time Bayes formula (equation 4) is iterated with a new clinical datum, the resultant probability $[P(D_i|C)]$ is called *posterior probability* of the diagnosis, replacing the prior probability at the next iteration. Accordingly, after the first iteration, the revised prior probability will no longer equal the prevalence, because the value of the prior probability changed, while that of the prevalence did not.

An expanded Bayes formula enables simultaneous processing of clinical data, instead of iterating the basic formula (equation 4) for each clinical datum.

$$P(D_i|C_1...C_n) = $$

$$= \frac{P(D_i) \times P(C_1|D_i) \times P(C_2|D_i) \times ... \times P(C_n|D_i)}{P(D_i) \times P(C_1|D_i) \times P(C_2|D_i) \times ... \times P(C_n|D_i) + ... + P(D_1) \times P(C_1|D_1) \times P(C_2|D_1) \times ... \times P(C_n|D_1) + P(D_m) \times P(C_1|D_m) \times P(C_2|D_m) \times ... \times P(C_n|D_m)}$$

Where: $P(D|C_1...C_n) = $ probability of disease $D_1...D_i...D_m$, given the clinical data $C_1...C_n$

$\quad P(D) \quad = $ prior probability of disease $D_1...D_i...D_m = $ prevalence of the disease

$\quad P(C|D) \quad = $ probability of clinical datum C, given disease D = sensitivity (S) of clinical datum C for disease D

Replacing each $P(C|D)$ by its equivalent S, according to equation 1:

$$P(Di|C_1...C_n) = \frac{P(D_i) \times S_{1i} \times ... \times S_{ni}}{P(D_i) \times S_{1i} \times ... \times S_{ni} + ... + P(D_1) \times S_{11} \times ... \times S_{n1} + ... + P(D_m) \times S_{1m} \times ... \times S_{nm}}$$

Where $S_1...S_n = $ sensitivities of the clinical data for the corresponding diseases

The result of applying this equation equals that obtained with laborious iteration of the basic Bayes formula for each clinical datum. In this equation, the prior probability remains unchanged and always equals the prevalence of the disease.

Bayes formula is commutative, meaning that clinical data of the same disease can be processed in any order, yielding identical result. This process parallels a physician's diagnostic approach.

$$*******************************$$

One should not confuse clinical datum positive predictive value and specificity. Specificity is defined as the fraction of patients without the disease which do not manifest the clinical datum:

$$\text{Specificity} = \frac{\text{patients with true negative datum}}{\text{all patients without disease}} = \frac{\text{patients with true negative datum}}{\text{patients with true negative datum} + \text{patients with false positive datum}}$$

In probabilistic notation:

Specificity = P ($\bar{C} \mid \bar{D}$) or 1 − P (C $\mid \bar{D}$)

Where: P = probability

  $\bar{C}$ = clinical datum absent

  | = given

  $\bar{D}$ = no disease

  C = clinical datum present

Specificity is not an element of our algorithm.

****

3. *Cost*

Cost is another index that is attached to each clinical datum. In our context it involves not only expense, but also risk and discomfort resulting from the required test or procedure. *Expense* is quantifiable in dollars or any other currency. *Risk* can be statistically quantified by outcomes of the procedure, although it also depends on operator skill. *Discomfort* is a subjective feeling that depends in part on the invasiveness of the procedure and in part on patient apprehension, although the latter can be controlled with sedation or anesthesia. Discomfort cannot be expressed as an exact numerical value, but only can be assigned an estimated qualitative level such as none, small, intermediate, or great. Expense, risk, and discomfort—like apples and oranges—cannot be arithmetically combined into an exact overall cost. However, expense and risk can be qualitatively expressed in levels similar to discomfort, to make the latter comparable to the former two. It is practical to consider the maximum qualitative level of expense, risk, and discomfort, as representative of overall cost level.

$$Cost = \max \text{ (expense, risk, discomfort)}$$

Because cost does not participate in the calculation of the probability of diagnoses, its inexactness is not critical; it is considered only when selecting the most suitable clinical datum next to investigate in the patient, as explained later.

We assign to each clinical datum one of four overall cost categories: no cost (clinical data typically obtained through medical history and physical examination), small cost (*e.g.*, obtained through routine laboratory analysis, ECG, and other ancillary studies), intermediate cost (*e.g.*, colonoscopy, lymph node excision biopsy), and great cost (*e.g.*, liver biopsy, laparotomy.)

Cost must be compared to the *benefit* expected to result from acquiring a clinical datum. Benefit has two components: a quantitative component and a qualitative component. The *quantitative component* depends on the positive predictive value (PP value) and sensitivity (S) of the clinical datum, which in turn determine the probability (P) of the corresponding diagnoses. PP value of a clinical datum present in a patient tends to increase the P of the corresponding diagnoses; S of a clinical datum absent tends to reduce the P of the corresponding diagnoses (page 32.) The clinical datum that has the greatest PP value or the greatest S will result in the greatest benefit because it increments the difference between the probability of the most likely diagnoses and the probabilities of those less likely, which are ultimately eliminated from the differential diagnosis list. The magnitude of the increment of the aforementioned difference of diagnostic probabilities quantifies the benefit of the clinical datum that produces it. The quantitative component of benefit can be determined before actually investigating a

29

clinical datum for presence or absence in the patient, by virtually testing with the algorithm both possible outcomes.

The *qualitative component* of benefit cannot be quantified; it depends on multiple factors such as patient health status and ability to tolerate the procedure, patient financial status, insurance company approval, prognosis, involved physician liability, and existence of efficacious and available treatments for the diseases listed in the differential diagnosis. Benefit must equal or exceed cost. The evaluation of cost-benefit of a clinical datum and the decision to implement a procedure to obtain it must be discussed with and approved by the patient. If the patient is wealthy, is not discouraged by the risk, or can tolerate discomfort, a procedure that incurs a greater cost may be acceptable. Confirmation of an uncertain diagnosis of a potentially life-threatening but treatable disease also may justify implementation of a more costly procedure.

Because cost and benefit cannot be accurately quantified, neither can cost-benefit ratio. If all of the aforementioned qualitative factors could be given an empiric value, it might be possible to devise an algorithm to assist the physician in better evaluating cost-benefit.

Summarizing how the three indices of clinical data—S, PP value, and cost—are determined: S depends on the clinical datum and corresponding disease; it is determined statistically with equation 2 (page 24.) PP value depends on S of the clinical datum for the disease under consideration and S of the same clinical datum for all diseases that manifest this datum; it is determined with equation 5 (page 26.) Cost—expense, risk, and discomfort—depends on the nature of the test or procedure needed to obtain the clinical datum; it is assigned one of four empirical categories: none, low, intermediate, or great.

Identifiers

Identifiers are assigned to a clinical datum when potentially dangerous circumstances prevail; they typically prompt a more extensive diagnostic work-up. A **risk identifier** flags any high-risk clinical datum (*e.g.*, dyspnea, chest pain, bleeding, laboratory test "panic" values) and any diagnosis with potentially bad outcome (*e.g.*, myocardial infarction, pulmonary embolism, malignancy.) An **interaction identifier** flags a clinical datum that might have been modified or masked by a drug interaction or a concurrent disease. Algorithms should check for such interactions. The use of identifiers will be explained later.

Before explaining how our algorithm relates to sensitivity, positive predictive value, and cost, we must discuss the ruling in and ruling out of diagnoses.

RULING IN AND RULING OUT DIAGNOSES

A diagnosis is *ruled in* when it is included in the differential diagnosis; this occurs whenever a patient clinical datum matches a clinical datum in the respective disease model.

A diagnosis is *ruled out* when it is deleted from the differential diagnosis; this occurs whenever the probability of the diagnosis falls below an empirical threshold. Clinical data that reduce the probability of a diagnosis favor the deletion of this diagnosis from the differential diagnosis.

These statements imply that a diagnosis must be ruled in before it can be ruled out.

When a new patient, for whom no clinical data are known comes to our attention, we consider two methods of achieving a final diagnosis:

The first method begins with a blank page—not knowing the patient's disease—and then formulating a differential diagnosis based on clinical data manifested by the patient. These patient clinical data, when matched with disease model clinical data, gradually increment the number of possible diagnoses; this process is called *ruling in diagnoses*. The greater PP value of a clinical datum that is *present*, the more likely the corresponding diagnosis. For example, microhemagglutination for *Treponema pallidum* test (MHA-TP) is a clinical datum of great PP value for syphilis; accordingly, if positive, it rules in this disease with great probability, because few other diseases manifest this clinical datum. A clinical datum that is present, with great PP value, strongly rules in the diagnosis, even if its S is small, meaning that this clinical datum is not frequently found, but as it is already present in this case, S is irrelevant. For example, filarias present in a blood sample is a clinical datum with great PP value for filariasis, confirming this diagnosis, despite a small S. On the other hand, a clinical datum present, typically would not favor a diagnosis only because it has a great S, because it simply tells that this clinical datum is frequently manifested by the specified disease, but many other diseases also may manifest it (small PP value). For example, weight loss has a great S for hyperthyroidism, but a small PP value; therefore, to rule in hyperthyroidism, a clinical datum with a greater PP value, such as suppressed thyroid stimulating hormone (TSH) must be investigated. A clinical datum that is present, with small S, typically would not rule in a diagnosis, because it simply means that this clinical datum is rare for the disease, which is not a reason *per se* to rule in the disease; for example, diarrhea (small S and small PP value) for duodenal ulcer. Accordingly, *ruling in a diagnosis relies on a clinical datum that is present and the greater its PP value the more it will support this diagnosis. S is irrelevant* if the clinical datum is present.

The second method of achieving a final diagnosis begins with all known diseases, gradually decrementing the number of possible diagnoses as sequentially investigated clinical data are found absent. An unknown patient could have *any* disease; for example, when we notice that he is a male, we realize that he cannot have an ovarian cancer; because he is young, prostate cancer is unlikely, and so forth. This process is called *ruling out* potential *diagnoses*. To *rule out* a potential diagnosis, we rely on the *sensitivity* of *clinical data* that are *absent* in the patient. The greater the S of a clinical datum that is absent, the less likely the corresponding diagnosis, even if the PP value is great, because the clinical datum is absent. For example, microhemagglutination test for *Treponema pallidum* (MHA-TP) is a clinical datum of great S for syphilis; accordingly, if negative, it rules out this disease because it is positive in essentially all cases of syphilis (rare false negative tests). As mentioned in the previous paragraph, weight loss is a clinical datum with great S for severe hyperthyroidism, because it is manifested in all such cases; accordingly, if this clinical datum is absent, this diagnosis tends to be ruled out. A clinical datum that is absent, with small S, has little influence on the probability of the diagnosis, even if PP value is great; for example, filarias negative in blood (great PP value, but small S) for filariasis. Small sensitivity of an absent clinical datum does not rule out the corresponding diagnosis because it only means that the clinical datum is rare for the disease; absence of a rare clinical datum does not exclude a diagnosis. For example diarrhea with small S and small PP value for duodenal ulcer, if absent, does not rule out this diagnosis. Accordingly, *ruling out a diagnosis relies on clinical data that are absent and with great S; PP value is irrelevant* if the clinical datum is absent.

This second method to achieve a final diagnosis is impractical because to analyze the several thousand known diseases would require a prohibitively large number of absent clinical data to rule out all but one or a few diseases. In reality, ruling in or ruling out is applied according to whether the clinical datum under consideration is present or absent, respectively. Essential rule:

A clinical datum present rules in the corresponding diagnosis with strength proportional to its positive predictive value (PP value). A clinical datum absent rules out the corresponding diagnosis with strength proportional to its sensitivity (S).

Table 2 shows how PP value and S of a clinical datum affect the P and ruling in or ruling out of a diagnosis according to whether the datum is present or absent in the patient.

Clinical datum	PP value	S	P	Effect on Diagnosis	Example	Comments
Present	Great	Great	Increased	Strongly ruled in	MHA-TP test for syphilis	Ruling in a diagnosis relies on clinical data present, with great PP value; S is irrelevant
	Great	Small	Increased	Strongly ruled in	Filariae in blood for filariasis	
	Small	Great	Unchanged	Weakly ruled in	Weight loss for hyperthyroidism	
	Small	Small	Unchanged	Weakly ruled in	Diarrhea for duodenal ulcer	
Absent	Great	Great	Decreased	Strongly ruled out	MHA-TP test for syphilis	Ruling out a diagnosis relies on clinical data absent, with great S; PP value is irrelevant
	Great	Small	Slightly changed according to value of S	Weakly ruled out	Filariae in blood for filariasis	
	Small	Great	Decreased	Strongly ruled out	Weight loss for hyperthyroidism	
	Small	Small	Slightly changed according to value of S	Weakly ruled out	Diarrhea for duodenal ulcer	

TABLE 2. MHA-TP, microhemagglutination for *Treponema palladium*, a highly exclusive and sensitive test for syphilis; PP value, positive predictive value; S, sensitivity; P, probability of diagnosis.

Eight combinations are possible—clinical datum present with great PP value, clinical datum present with great S, clinical datum present with small PP value, clinical datum present with small S, clinical datum absent with great PP value, clinical datum absent with great S, clinical datum absent with small PP value, and clinical datum absent with small S. Of these eight combinations, only two are useful—clinical datum present with great PP value and clinical datum absent with great S—because only they can significantly change the P of the corresponding diagnosis; all other combinations are discarded.

OPERATION OF OUR DIAGNOSTIC ALGORITHM

I. INITIAL CLINICAL DATA COLLECTION

The diagnostic process begins with collection of initial clinical data gleaned from the patient's history, physical examination, and prior consultations. These *initial* clinical data, entered in the computer, are unrefined because we do not yet know their PP value nor S. Each of these values depend on the clinical datum collected, but also on the corresponding, but as yet not ruled in diagnosis. Initially, collection is focused primarily on clinical data present because only these can rule in diagnoses. At this early phase, clinical data processing is purely categorical because we have not yet applied any probabilistic calculations; the diagnostic process is called *ill structured* [24]. Only after potential diagnoses are selected can S and PP value of clinical data be determined, the P of each diagnosis be calculated, and a differential diagnosis list be created; the diagnostic process then is said to be *well structured*. Then, if warranted, diagnoses can be ruled out by processing clinical data absent.

How many clinical data to collect?

Ideally and theoretically, to avoid missing a patient's disease, all existing clinical data (several thousand) should be investigated for presence or absence in every patient. Realistically speaking, this is impossible because of time and cost restrictions; it would kill every patient and the socioeconomic system. Were it possible to do such a search, the diagnostic process would probably become totally categorical and logical eliminating any guesswork concerning probability estimates. Because time and financial resources are limited, we are forced to do an imperfect diagnostic job. Statistics, probabilities, and heuristics will help us to bridge the gaps. This takes health care providers into an inexact arena where liability lurks, even for the most talented and well intentioned.

How can we reconcile these two opposing forces, namely gathering sufficient medical information *versus* time and cost restrictions? A perfect solution does not exist, but heuristic methods became handy. We begin by collecting all possible no cost clinical data that are obtainable from the history and physical examination, and perhaps from the low cost ancillary tests. Later on, we will describe and utilize heuristic restrictive methods (*e.g.*, best cost-benefit clinical datum next to investigate) to avoid the collection of futile clinical data. Algorithms can be provided with safeguard identifiers that preclude incomplete or incorrect diagnoses. One routine may search for risk identifiers associated with specific *clinical data* implying serious diagnoses, and assures that these data are not overlooked by the diagnostic process. Another routine may search for risk identifiers associated with *diagnoses* that imply serious diseases and assures that these diagnoses are included in the differential diagnosis list. Still another routine searches for clinical entities potentially related to the *final diagnosis*, such as causes or complications, and include them in the differential diagnosis to be confirmed or ruled out. Watchful deferral of diagnoses, empirical treatment, and diagnosis by exclusion, are additional useful heuristic methods, to be described later.

Despite safeguards that preclude overlooking diseases, we still could miss an asymptomatic disease such as dyslipdemia, mild diabetes, or incipient cancer in an ostensibly healthy patient, were we not to carry out the early disease detection tests (page 19.)

Two alternative methods exist for collecting and processing clinical data:

Comprehensive method

The comprehensive method collects as many no cost and small cost clinical data as possible; these are obtained from the history and physical examination and perhaps some ancillary studies (as mentioned in "Health Assessment and Early Detection of Disease" on page 19.) This approach includes clinical data manifested by both apparent and occasionally asymptomatic diseases. We prefer this method because the algorithm emulates traditional physician processing of comprehensive initial information, thereby reducing the risk that the algorithm would arrive at an incomplete or even incorrect diagnosis, as exemplified by the abridged method described in the next paragraph.

Abridged method

The abridged method begins with the patient's chief complaint, then gradually refines the diagnostic process by investigating new clinical data recommended by the algorithm. The *chief complaint* is a symptom (*e.g.*, chest pain) or sign (*e.g.*, bleeding) that prompts the patient to seek medical attention. Accordingly, it might be convenient, although not mandatory, to begin the diagnostic process with the chief complaint; if the patient manifests other significant clinical data, they can be processed at the same time. This abridged, managed-care-style medical examination risks overlooking concurrent occult diseases, arriving at an incomplete or incorrect diagnosis. Should the patient's clinical status be unknown (*e.g.*, first visit or patient not seen recently), an urgent follow-up appointment for a complete history and physical examination is mandated as outlined in section "Health Assessment and Early Detection of Disease" (page 19.) Examples of how insufficient clinical data can lead to an incomplete or incorrect diagnosis are:

- **Incomplete diagnosis**: dyspnea, distal edema, bibasal pulmonary rales, hepatomegaly, and cardiac gallop rhythm are the clinical data provided to the computer. Without additional information, the algorithm would correctly diagnose congestive heart failure syndrome. The algorithm might conclude that this syndromic diagnosis is the only final diagnosis, overlooking its underlying cause (*e.g.*, myocardial infarction). This would be even more likely if the chest pain of myocardial infarction is masked by concurrent diabetes. Such an incomplete diagnosis could have dismal consequences because treatment primarily should be directed against the cause and secondarily against the resulting syndrome.

- **Incorrect diagnosis**: headache, fever, vomiting, photophobia, and neck rigidity are the clinical data provided to the computer. An experienced physician would immediately recognize this constellation of clinical data as characteristic of meningitis even before performing a detailed history and physical examination (this is called the "clinical eye".) The algorithm processes sequentially the first clinical data as they are provided (*e.g.*, headache, fever, and vomiting) and might prematurely conclude an incorrect final diagnosis (*e.g.*, acute gastritis), before requesting more characteristic data (*e.g.*, neck rigidity). Initially providing the algorithm with all possible no cost and small cost clinical data appears to enable an earlier and better-structured differential diagnosis.

Our algorithm applies the *all-inclusive method* to integrate a differential diagnosis list (page 37), which includes in the differential diagnosis list all the diagnoses evoked by all the clinical data initially collected with the *comprehensive method*, rendering unnecessary to specifically check for risk flagged diagnoses and clinical data. We mention risks flagged clinical data and diagnoses only as a convenient precaution for other researchers to preclude overlooking dangerous diseases when creating algorithms that are not based on the mentioned methods.

In spite of the above considerations, it is still unclear whether the abridged method would provide the shortest and most economic path to a correct final diagnosis, or request inappropriately numerous, time consuming and costly clinical data in an effort to obtain the missing information to achieve this diagnosis. Testing both comprehensive and abridged methods with actual clinical cases can clarify these uncertainties. Essential rule:

A diagnostic algorithm must neither miss correct diagnoses nor recommend inappropriate or unnecessarily costly clinical data.

II. SELECTING POTENTIAL DIAGNOSES

Following initial clinical data collection (page 33), the algorithm next must compare each clinical datum manifested by the patient with all clinical data listed in all disease models stored in the knowledge base, selecting those disease models that contain one or more matching clinical data. Such disease models represent potential diagnoses that will become the differential diagnosis list. As mentioned on page 14, this task involves important difficulties that are, in my opinion, a major reason why a satisfactory diagnostic algorithm has not yet been achieved:

- A disease typically never manifests all clinical data listed in its disease model.

- The cost of obtaining some of these clinical data may be prohibitive.

- Diverse diseases can manifest similar clinical data; in other words, most clinical data are not pathognomonic.

- After selection of potential diagnoses, the algorithm must establish whether they are *competing* for a single final diagnosis or whether they correspond to *concurrent* diseases. Essential rule:

An efficient algorithm must distinguish competing diagnoses from concurrent diseases.

Later on we will explain how our algorithm deals with these problems.

We encounter here the semantic problem discussed on page 13: when should we use the term diagnosis and when disease? In this context the difference between these two terms is blurred because we are in a field between the patient's physical reality (disease) and the physician's mental perception of this reality (diagnosis).

III. CLINICAL DATUM LISTS

Having selected the matching disease models that now represent potential diagnoses, the algorithm creates, for each clinical datum present, a list that has for heading this clinical datum and comprises all potential diagnoses able to manifest such clinical datum.

A CLINICAL DATUM LIST is a list of diagnoses (*e.g.*, bronchitis, asthma, lung cancer) that a single clinical datum (*e.g.*, cough) evokes in the mind of the physician, which is analogous to the matching of a single clinical datum with clinical data in disease models by the computer. Such diagnoses, as opposed to diseases, are in the mind of the physician; the patient is not afflicted by all of them. Each of these *potential diagnoses* has a probability to become a *final diagnosis*, the latter ideally being concordant with the disease that afflicts the patient. A proper denomination for clinical datum list would be **Potential diagnoses list for a single clinical datum**, which is lengthy and cumbersome. For that reason, we abbreviate it to **Clinical datum list**, because despite being a list of diagnoses, the clinical datum identifies the list and is its heading.

Clinical datum list should not be mistaken with disease model, which has a disease as its heading and lists **all** clinical data that this disease can manifest.

Clinical datum
Matching disease model → Potential diagnosis 1
Matching disease model → Potential diagnosis 2

      ⋮   ⋮

Matching disease model → Potential diagnosis n

The sensitivity (S) and positive predictive value (PP value) of the clinical datum for each potential diagnosis is shown. The diagnoses are sorted by decreasing PP value. In addition, a risk identifier flags clinical data and diagnoses that involve great risk or bad prognosis (not necessary for our algorithm; see page 34), and an interaction identifier flags clinical data that may be modified by drugs or concurrent diseases (page 30). Examples of clinical datum lists are:

Hemoptysis	S	PP value
(bleeding from respiratory tract)		
Tuberculosis	0.70	0.35 *
Lung cancer	0.40	0.20
Lung infarction	0.30	0.15
Bronchitis	0.05	0.025
Pneumonia	0.03	0.015
⋮	⋮	⋮

Dyspnea (difficulty to breathe)	S	PP value
Asthma	0.98	0.208
Congestive heart failure	0.80	0.17
Foreign body aspiration	0.80	0.17
Pneumonia	0.40	0.085
Emphysema	0.39	0.083
Carbon monoxide intoxication	0.22	0.047
Lung cancer	0.20	0.042
Lung infarction	0.19	0.04
Tuberculosis	0.17	0.036
Intense anemia	0.12	0.025
⋮	⋮	⋮

Cough	S	PP value
Foreign body aspiration	1.00	0.20
Bronchitis	0.98	0.196
Tuberculosis	0.70	0.14
Lung cancer	0.50	0.10
Lung infarction	0.40	0.08
Pneumonia	0.20	0.04
⋮	⋮	⋮

*   The numeric values for S and PP value in the above examples were not obtained from actual statistics or calculations. Cost, risk and interaction identifiers were omitted for the sake of simplicity.

In a complete clinical datum list, the sum of the PP values equals 1. The fewer diagnoses a clinical datum list comprises, the more the clinical datum supports those diagnoses and the greater the corresponding PP values. When a clinical datum list contains only one diagnosis, PP value = 1, meaning the clinical datum is exclusive or pathognomonic for this diagnosis. Conversely, the more diagnoses a clinical datum list comprises, the less the clinical datum supports those diagnoses, and the smaller their corresponding PP values.

IV. DIFFERENTIAL DIAGNOSIS LIST

This step creates a *differential diagnosis list* that comprises potential diagnoses transferred from the clinical datum lists.

Here again, we have a semantic problem: a suitable name for DIFFERENTIAL DIAGNOSIS LIST could be **Potential diagnoses list for more than one clinical datum** manifested by a patient. This denomination is long and cumbersome; we could abbreviate it to **Potential diagnoses list**, but because DIFFERENTIAL DIAGNOSIS LIST is customary we retained the latter. Do not mistake clinical datum list with differential diagnosis list.

How many diagnoses should be included in the differential diagnosis list?

Several sections of this research pose problems that admit diverse solutions. Our preferred methods —that we consider simple, elegant, and practical—to solve these problems are strongly supported by manual calculations and results.

Diverse methods can be followed regarding which of all the diagnoses brought up in the entire set of clinical datum lists should be included in the differential diagnosis list. Our algorithm functions properly only with the all-inclusive method described below.

All-inclusive method to integrate a differential diagnosis list

This method is **essential** to validate further routines involved in our algorithm. It includes in the differential diagnosis list *all diagnoses* listed in all clinical datum lists, without repeating similar diagnoses; in other words, all the potential diagnoses brought up thus far.

This method generates a relatively long differential diagnosis list and involves the burden of investigating the presence or absence of clinical data related to each diagnosis. However, this burden is not problematic because this method is applied at an early diagnostic stage when collected initial clinical data are already known to be present or absent, and the number of matched diagnoses is not excessive. Later, heuristically restrictive tools such as the best cost-benefit clinical datum next to investigate (page 53) will further limit proliferation of clinical data and diagnoses.

Were we from the beginning to use the comprehensive method for collecting and processing as many no cost clinical data as possible (page 34) we would be less likely to miss a diagnosis. At the same time, we would avoid excessive proliferation of information because these more numerous clinical data are likely to include a clinical datum that confirms a final diagnosis, rendering unnecessary further searching.

The all-inclusive method renders unnecessary the risk identifiers (page 30), because it includes automatically both risk and non-risk diagnoses in the differential diagnosis list.

Example of all-inclusive method generating a long differential diagnosis list: an 18-year-old female presented with fever peaking to 40° C for several months (an actual case from my private practice); the history and physical examination otherwise were completely normal during the entire course of the disease. Hundreds of tests, from the simplest to the most sophisticated, yielded normal results. Several specialists at a prestigious university medical center were consulted, without achieving a final diagnosis; this was a genuine case of fever of unknown origin. Several months later, the fever spontaneously resolved and the patient remained healthy during several months of follow up. In this case, the differential diagnosis list is identical to the clinical datum list for fever, because the patient did not manifest any other clinical datum. An exhaustive diagnostic work up, searching for additional clinical data, was needed because the parsimony principle (next paragraphs, alternative methods) is not applicable to a single clinical datum. The diagnoses that can account for fever are numerous. The more the diagnoses comprised by a single clinical datum list the less exclusive the clinical datum; the PP value for each diagnosis is small, because the sum of all the PP values of these diagnoses must total 1. Accordingly, the single clinical datum of fever cannot significantly increase the P of any of these diagnoses. The final diagnosis must be supported by other more exclusive clinical data, with greater PP value. The small PP value of a clinical datum gains importance when no other clinical datum with greater PP value is available; in such cases competing diagnoses must be ruled-out with absent clinical data of great sensitivity (S). This issue is related to the diagnosis by exclusion (page 91.) In our example, essentially all diagnoses were ruled out, without confirming any.

The following alternative methods are discussed only for historical reasons, but in our opinion are inaccurate and do not function with some further steps of our algorithm.

Majority method to integrate a differential diagnosis list

The majority method includes in the differential diagnosis list only *diagnoses supported by the majority of manifested clinical data* (*i.e., listed in the majority of clinical datum lists.*) The rationale here is that each such diagnosis can account for all or most clinical data so far manifested by the patient. To consider a single diagnosis that accounts for all manifested clinical data is simpler than considering two or more diagnoses. This satisfies the principle of parsimony (also called unitary hypothesis or Occam's razor principle) that favors the simplest of several solutions. However, were a single final diagnosis not to account for all manifested clinical data, a search for concurrent disease that account for the remaining clinical data would be mandated. The parsimony principle limits the number of diagnoses in the differential diagnosis list, but increases the risk of missing concurrent disease.

Example of majority method that overlooks an important diagnosis, but the risk identifier of this diagnosis is recognized by the algorithm and the diagnosis is included in the differential diagnosis list. A patient presents with bright red fecal blood and varicose hemorrhoidal veins, pointing to a final diagnosis of bleeding hemorrhoids, a frequent disease that accounts for the obtained clinical data. Less frequently, concurrent colorectal cancer also manifests fecal blood; in this case the hemorrhoidal disease is a red herring that can cause cancer to be overlooked. However, because in the *fecal blood* clinical datum list, *colorectal cancer* is risk-flagged, the algorithm includes this diagnosis in the differential diagnosis list. Then, the algorithm's best cost-benefit clinical datum function looks for the clinical datum with the greatest PP value for colorectal cancer, which is an endoscopy and biopsy (PP value = 1) that when positive confers a P = 1, confirming this diagnosis.

Example of majority method aborted by parsimony principle. A patient presents with fever, sore throat, and whitish exudate covering both pharyngeal tonsils yielding a positive culture for Group A β-hemolytic streptococcus. The diagnosis of streptococcal tonsillitis accounts for all of the mentioned clinical data. Supported by the parsimony principle, few clinicians would further pursue this case with such an obvious diagnosis.

Probability method to integrate a differential diagnosis list

The probability method includes in the differential diagnosis list only *diagnoses of great probability* (P), even when they do not account for all or most of the patient's clinical data; this alternative also is based on the parsimony principle. In actual clinical cases perhaps no difference exists between a diagnosis that accounts for all clinical data and the most probable diagnosis, because that diagnosis would fulfil both conditions; if so, no major difference exists between majority and probability methods. A diagnosis that accounts for most of a patient's clinical data might only *suggest* a final diagnosis that would then need to be validated by great probability (P).

The majority and probability methods have the disadvantage of sometimes wrongfully discarding a diagnosis that accounts for only a few clinical data or a diagnosis with a small P. At this point, such a diagnosis might represent only the "tip of the iceberg," especially when only a few clinical data are collected. When additional clinical data of great PP value supporting such a diagnosis are found present, the number of existing clinical data rationalized by this diagnosis or the probability of this diagnosis might increase remarkably.

In an attempt to preclude wrongfully discarding diagnoses when the majority or the probability method is used, the algorithm checks for risk-flagged diagnoses in the clinical datum lists and for clinical entities linked to final diagnoses, then includes all of them in the differential diagnosis list to be processed. However, cases with atypical evolution, delayed resolution, or difficult diagnosis warrant application of the all-inclusive method.

Example of shortcoming of majority and probability methods: same patient as in the previous example, presenting with fever, sore throat, and whitish exudate covering both pharyngeal tonsils that is culture-positive for Group A β-hemolytic streptococcus. In this case, a 10-day antibiotic treatment course did not resolve the symptoms. Suspecting the tonsillitis might be caused by some other disease, the clinician decided to pursue a more comprehensive work up. He must switch from these methods to our essential one, including in the differential diagnosis list all the remaining diagnoses included in the clinical datum lists fever, sore throat, tonsillar exudate, and streptococcus. Notice that the identified bacterium has a great PP value, although less than 1, because it *could* merely be an innocent bystander (asymptomatic streptococcus carrier status includes about 20% of the general population.) The best cost-benefit clinical datum function will recommend the investigation of clinical data such as lymph node swellings in areas other than the neck, heterophile antibody test, CBC, splenomegaly, and signs of hepatitis, leading the physician towards the originally unsuspected diagnosis of infectious mononucleosis.

V. PROBABILITY OF DIAGNOSES. MINI-MAX PROCEDURE

At this point we have a well-structured diagnostic problem with a differential diagnosis list. Next, the algorithm must determine which of these potential diagnoses will become one or more final diagnoses.

My son Tomás Feder, a computer scientist, helped me devise a procedure for calculating the probability (P) of a diagnosis by combining the PP value of clinical data when *present* (favoring a diagnosis) with the S of clinical data when *absent* (disfavoring a diagnosis). We call it the *mini-max procedure**. In successive steps, we will explain this procedure with examples.

* Our term mini-max is reminiscent of a similar term used in game theory, but not previously applied in combination with Bayes formula to calculate probability of diagnoses.

Step 1. Process clinical data present

To establish the value of P, other diagnostic programs add, subtract, multiply, or average the sensitivities, specificities, predictive values, estimated values of clinical data supporting a diagnosis, or iterate Bayes formula with each additional clinical datum. These approaches have flaws.

For example, jaundice, dark urine, and increased direct serum bilirubin are clinical data related by similar pathophysiologic mechanisms generated by a single lesion: biliary tract obstruction. Were we arithmetically to combine the individual PP values of these three equivalent and "redundant" clinical data, P of diagnosis biliary tract obstruction would be improperly increased thereby providing an undue advantage to this diagnosis, as compared to competing diagnoses. Furthermore, assume that an endoscopic retrograde cholangiopancreatography (ERCP) shows a biliary stone obstructing the common bile duct —a clinical datum that alone has a confirmatory PP value of 1. If we add the PP values of other supporting clinical data, the P of the diagnosis obstructing gallstones would exceed 1, which is probabilistically impossible. If we average or multiply these PP values, the confirmatory PP value 1 would be unduly reduced.

With our algorithm, the PP value of gallstone obstruction, which equals 1, supersedes all other clinical data with smaller PP value (jaundice, dark urine, increased serum bilirubin) because—whether present or absent—they would not change the diagnosis of obstructing gallstones already confirmed by ERCP.

Accordingly, we consider that the greatest PP value of these related clinical data better represents the P of the diagnosis than any arithmetical combination of the individual values. Essential rule:

The probability (P) of a diagnosis equals the greatest positive predictive value (PP value) of the clinical data that support this diagnosis.

For each diagnosis in the differential diagnosis list, the algorithm looks in the entire set of clinical datum lists and selects the greatest PP value that supports *this* diagnosis. The selected greatest PP value equals the P of this diagnosis.

$$P = \max (PP \text{ value}_1 \dots PP \text{ value}_n) \tag{6}$$

Where P = probability of the diagnosis under consideration

max = maximum of

PP value $_1$… PP value $_n$ = positive predictive values of clinical data present, that support the diagnosis under consideration

The algorithm then iterates the same routine to determine the P of each diagnosis in the differential diagnosis list.

Example: a patient presents with cough, hemoptysis, dyspnea, expectoration, and *Mycobacterium tuberculosis* (*Mycobacterium TB*) in sputum. Five clinical datum lists are generated:

Cough	S	PP value
Pulmonary tuberculosis	0.80	0.276
Pulmonary embolism	0.50	0.172
Bronchiectasis	0.90	0.310
Lung cancer	0.70	0.241

Hemoptysis	S	PP value
Pulmonary tuberculosis	0.40	0.222
Pulmonary embolism	0.60	0.333
Bronchiectasis	0.30	0.167
Lung cancer	0.50	0.278

Dyspnea	S	PP value
Pulmonary tuberculosis	0.20	0.148
Pulmonary embolism	0.50	0.370
Bronchiectasis	0.05	0.037
Lung cancer	0.60	0.444

Expectoration	S	PP value
Pulmonary tuberculosis	0.80	0.417
Pulmonary embolism	0.02	0.010
Bronchiectasis	0.90	0.469
Lung cancer	0.20	0.104

Mycobacterium TB	S	PP value
Pulmonary tuberculosis	0.70	1.000
Pulmonary embolism	0.00	0.000
Bronchiectasis	0.00	0.000
Lung cancer	0.00	0.000

S values in the above example are for demonstration purposes only and do not represent actual statistics. PP values were calculated by applying equation 5 (page 26) to these S values. We assume that only the four listed diagnoses exist and that any of them could account for the five clinical data. Highlighted values refer to clinical data that are not elements of a specific disease model; accordingly, their S and PP value values equal 0. Such clinical data have no influence on calculated probabilities.

In the entire set of clinical datum lists, the greatest PP value for pulmonary tuberculosis is 1.000 and equals P for this diagnosis. Similarly, 0.370 for pulmonary embolism, 0.469 for brochiectasis, and 0.444 for lung cancer.

A differential diagnosis list is created, with each diagnosis showing the respective P that competes with the P of the other diagnoses for a final diagnosis. The diagnoses are sorted by decreasing P values.

Differential diagnosis list	P
Pulmonary tuberculosis	1.000
Bronchiectasis	0.469
Lung cancer	0.444
Pulmonary embolism	0.370

Except for confirmed pulmonary tuberculosis, these P values do not yet satisfy thresholds that enable to rule out the other diagnoses or confirm some as concurrent final diagnosis (how such thresholds are determined will be explained later on page 87.) To satisfy this threshold requirement, the algorithm automatically determines which additional best cost-benefit clinical datum (page 53) should next be investigated for its presence or absence. Fever is first recommended for investigation, followed by a pulmonary cavity lesion:

Fever	S	PP value	Cavity	S	PP value
Pulmonary tuberculosis	0.70	0.636	Pulmonary tuberculosis	0.60	0.600
Pulmonary embolism	0.30	0.273	Pulmonary embolism	0.00	0.000
Bronchiectasis	0.00	0.000	Bronchiectasis	0.10	0.100
Lung cancer	0.10	0.091	Lung cancer	0.30	0.300

Were fever and a pulmonary cavity lesion also *present* in the patient, we would now have a total of seven clinical datum lists. Were the PP value associated with any of the diagnoses in these 2 new clinical datum lists to exceed the P of the same diagnosis, that greater PP value would replace this existing P.

PP value of a clinical datum present can only **increase** the probability of a diagnosis (equation 6, page 40.)

Step 2. Process clinical data absent

Only those clinical data absent that are related to diagnoses in the differential diagnosis list are processed.

We presented a rational explanation and example of why we believe that the greatest PP value of all the clinical data *present* that supports a specific diagnosis equals the P of this diagnosis. This is consequent to the fact that clinical data present are related by a common lesion or cause; adding the PP values of these clinical data would excessively increase this P. On page 31, we discussed how the sensitivity (S) of a clinical datum *absent* typically reduces the P of the corresponding diagnosis. To reduce P of the corresponding diagnosis, some authors arithmetically combine S of all absent clinical data, or sequentially apply Bayes formula to each S of such clinical data. We observed that this procedure excessively decreases the P of the diagnosis to a value that might incorrectly rule out the corresponding disease. For this reason, to reduce the P of a diagnosis, we use only the greatest S of all clinical data absent. This approach for disfavoring a diagnosis is less intuitive than using the greatest PP value of clinical data present for supporting a diagnosis. Clinical data absent are not related by a common lesion or cause; however, they might be related by a specific characteristic of patient's body that is responsible for the failure to react, or the cause is insufficient to evoke all potential clinical data. This common denominator justifies considering only the datum absent of greatest S as the representative of all clinical data absent. The following example supports this approach:

Consider again a patient with a suspected common bile duct obstruction by gallstones. An endoscopic retrograde cholangiopancreatography (ERCP) in this case was negative—*i.e.*, *no* gallstones were present in the common bile duct, an absent clinical datum of great S (close to 1) for the mentioned diagnosis. To rule out this diagnosis, it is unnecessary to consider additional clinical data absent of smaller S, such as right upper abdominal pain or vomiting.

So far, we have explained how clinical data present and their associated PP values determine the P of a diagnosis. Now we will explain how clinical data absent and their associated S values further influence this P. Originally, we tried this equation:

$$P = PP \text{ value} \times (1-S) \tag{7}$$

Where PP value = probability of a diagnosis **before** considering the sensitivity of a clinical datum absent; this probability equals the greatest PP value of all clinical data present that support this diagnosis (equation 6, page 40)

   P = probability of this diagnosis **after** considering the S of a clinical datum absent pertaining to the same diagnosis

   S = sensitivity of a clinical datum absent pertaining to the same diagnosis.

With equation 7, the greater the S of a clinical datum absent, the more it reduces the P of a diagnosis.

Let's assume that fever and cavity in a previous example, were investigated and found *absent* and let's apply equation 7. *Mycobacterium tuberculosis* was found in the sputum, a clinical datum present with a PP value = 1, which confers a P = 1 to tuberculosis, confirming this diagnosis. Next, our example considers fever, a clinical datum absent with S = 0.7. Applying equation 7, we obtain:

$$P = PP \text{ value} \times (1-S) = 1 \times (1-0.7) = 0.3$$

Notice that the absence of fever decreases tuberculosis P from 1 to 0.3. It is unacceptable that a relatively unimportant clinical datum absent, such as fever, should cause a substantial decrease in P, which tends to rule out the already confirmed diagnosis of tuberculosis.

To temper this unacceptable decrease in P caused by equation 7, we instead use:

$$\text{PP value}_i \, (1-S_i)$$
$$P_i$$

PP value$_1$…PP value$_i$…PP value$_n$ = positive predictive value of the same clinical datum present (*Mycobacterium tuberculosis* in sputum) for each respective diagnosis in the differential diagnosis list (4 diagnoses per our example)

S_1…S_i…S_n = sensitivity of the clinical datum absent (fever) for each respective diagnosis in the differential diagnosis list (4 diagnoses per our example)

Notice that the numerator of equation 8 is identical to the right member of equation 7, and that a denominator has been introduced, the effect of which is to "temper" the result. This denominator comprises several terms, each of which refers to a diagnosis in the differential diagnosis list. Each comprises the PP value of the clinical datum present (*Mycobacterium tuberculosis*) and the S of the clinical datum absent (fever). These clinical data present and absent remain *unchanged for all terms*; but their respective PP values and S values change to values associated with each diagnosis. Equation 7 is then applied to these values in each denominator term of equation 8.

Equation 8 is related to Bayes formula, but is here used differently than in other programs; it involves two clinical data supposedly *independent*—one present and the other absent. Accordingly, Bayes condition of independence is not violated.

Referring to our example of *Mycobacterium tuberculosis* present in sputum and fever absent, we now must apply equation 8 to calculate the probability of tuberculosis (P_{TB}):

$$P_{TB} = \frac{\text{PP value}_{TB}\,(1-S_{TB})}{\text{PPvalue}_{TB}(1-S_{TB})+\text{PPvalue}_{bronchiectasis}(1-S_{bronchiectasis})+\text{PPvalue}_{cancer}(1-S_{cancer})+\text{PPvalue}_{embolism}(1-S_{embolism})}$$

Substituting PP value and S with values from the clinical datum lists on pages 40 and 41, we obtain:

$$P_{TB} = \frac{1.00\,(1-0.70)}{1.00\,(1-0.70) + 0.00\,(1-0.00) + 0.00\,(1-0.10) + 0.00\,(1-0.30)} =$$

$$= \frac{0.30}{0.30 + 0.00 + 0.00 + 0.00} = 1.00$$

Notice that equation 8 retains the correct value of P = 1 for confirmed tuberculosis, instead of P = 0.30, as was obtained with equation 7.

Equation 8 yields identical result if all PP values of the clinical datum *present* are substituted with the corresponding S of the same clinical datum, S otherwise typically used with clinical data *absent*:

$$P_i = \frac{\text{PP value}_i\,(1-S_i)}{\text{PP value}_1\,(1-S_1) + … + \text{PP value}_i\,(1-S_i) + … + \text{PP value}_n\,(1-S_n)} = \frac{S_i\,(1-S_i)}{S_1\,(1-S_1) + … + S_i\,(1-S_i) + … + S_n\,(1-S_n)}$$

Notice that the value of S (sensitivity of the clinical datum *present*) is *not* the same as the value of S (sensitivity of the clinical datum *absent*). Equation 8, with PP values, yields identical result as with S because PP value and S of a given clinical datum for a given diagnosis are directly proportional. When all PP values are substituted with the right member of equation 5 (page 26), equation 8 can be simplified to its substituted form (right member) shown above. This simplification is possible because the sum $S_1+\ldots+S_i+\ldots+S_n$ in the numerator and denominator of equation 8 have identical values and cancel each other.

The denominator of equation 8—modified Bayes formula—can be seen as a *weighted average* of S of a clinical datum present for diverse diseases, weighted by S values of the clinical datum absent. Comparing the S of the clinical datum present for a specific disease with the average of S values for all diseases indicates the relative significance of the clinical datum for this specific disease.

For clarity and consistency, we will retain the original equation 8 (with PP values) for all further calculations, but the substituted form (with S values) might be useful for computer programming.

Equation 8 is then iterated to calculate the P that the clinical data pair *Mycobacterium tuberculosis*-fever confers to the remaining diagnoses in the differential diagnosis list. PP value and S value corresponding to each diagnosis must be substituted in the numerator; the denominator remains unchanged. Equation 8 *normalizes* the probabilities of the diagnoses, meaning that their sum ($P_{TB} + P_{bronchiectasis} + P_{cancer} + P_{embolism}$) now equals 1. Referring to our example:

Mycobacterium TB - **Fever**	**PP value**	**S**		**P**
Pulmonary tuberculosis	$1.000 \times (1\text{-}0.70) = 0.300$ (numerator)	$\div\ 0.300$ (denominator)	$= 1.000$
Pulmonary embolism	$0.000 \times (1\text{-}0.30) = 0.000$ (numerator)	$\div\ 0.300$ (denominator)	$= 0.000$
Bronchiectasis	$0.000 \times (1\text{-}0.00) = 0.000$ (numerator)	$\div\ 0.300$ (denominator)	$= 0.000$
Lung cancer	$0.000 \times (1\text{-}0.10) = 0.000$ (numerator)	$\div\ 0.300$ (denominator)	$= 0.000$
	Sum $= 0.300$ (denominator)		Sum $= 1.000$

Normalization

In this publication, normalization is used with two different meanings: (1) In data base organization it means transforming networks into tables and vice versa (page 94.) (2) In our probabilistic context, normalization means transformation of a set of values into a set of probabilities that sum 1, maintaining the original proportion among them, yielding compatible and comparable probabilities on a percentage base.

This takes us from the field of mere proportions into the realm of probability, where values are comprised between 0—event impossible—and 1—event certain. Between 0 and 1 is the uncertainty range where the probability of the event, in this case the correctness of a diagnosis (or a disease truly afflicting a patient) is a fraction of certainty 1. This is expressed in Bayes formula for *competing* diagnoses, and in its derived equations 5 and 8.

$$a + b + c = x \text{ is normalized to } \frac{a}{a+b+c} + \frac{b}{a+b+c} + \frac{c}{a+b+c} = 1$$

Where a, b, and c are sensitivities S in equation 5 and terms PP value $(1–S)$ in equation 8.

Step 3. Create clinical data pairs

As remarked above, equation 8 comprises a clinical datum present and a clinical datum absent; we call this clinical data combination a *clinical data pair*. Each clinical data pair confers a *partial probability* to a diagnosis. To calculate the *total probability* (page 46) of each diagnosis, the mini-max procedure must create *all possible clinical data pairs* with all thus-far investigated clinical data present and absent. The number of clinical data pairs created will equal the number of clinical data present multiplied by the number of clinical data absent.

Returning to our previous example, we had 5 clinical data present (cough, expectoration, hemoptysis, dyspnea, and *Mycobacterium tuberculosis*) and 2 clinical data absent (cavity and fever), creating a total of 10 clinical data pairs (cough-cavity, cough-fever, hemoptysis-cavity, hemoptysis-fever, dyspnea-cavity, dyspnea-fever, expectoration-cavity, expectoration-fever, *Mycobacterium tuberculosis*-cavity, and *Mycobacterium tuberculosis*-fever.)

Because PP value and S value vary with each diagnosis, the total number of resulting *partial P values* equal the number of clinical data pairs created multiplied by the number of diagnoses in the differential diagnosis list. In our example, we had 10 clinical data pairs and 4 diagnoses (pulmonary tuberculosis, pulmonary embolism, bronchiectasis, and lung cancer), yielding a total of 40 partial P values.

Step 4. Create clinical data pair tables

We then organize the 40 partial P values as 10 *clinical data pair tables*, one table for each clinical data pair. Each table is headed by the clinical data pair; its first column lists the diagnoses in the differential diagnosis list; intermediate columns apply equation 8, and its last column lists the resultant partial P values. For our example:

Clinical data pair tables

Cough-Cavity	**PP value**		S					**Partial P**
Pulmonary tuberculosis	0.276	×	(1-0.60)	=	0.110	÷	0.730	= 0.151
Pulmonary embolism	0.172	×	(1-0.00)	=	0.172	÷	0.730	= 0.236
Brochiectasis	0.310	×	(1-0.10)	=	0.279	÷	0.730	= 0.382
Lung cancer	0.241	×	(1-0.30)	=	0.169	÷	0.730	= 0.231
							0.730	1.000

Cough-Fever								
Pulmonary tuberculosis	0.276	×	(1-0.70)	=	0.083	÷	0.731	= 0.113
Pulmonary embolism	0.172	×	(1-0.30)	=	0.121	÷	0.731	= 0.165
Brochiectasis	0.310	×	(1-0.00)	=	0.310	÷	0.731	= 0.425
Lung cancer	0.241	×	(1-0.10)	=	0.217	÷	0.731	= 0.297
							0.731	1.000

Hemoptysis-Cavity								
Pulmonary tuberculosis	0.222	×	(1-0.60)	=	0.089	÷	0.767	= 0.116
Pulmonary embolism	0.333	×	(1-0.00)	=	0.333	÷	0.767	= 0.435
Brochiectasis	0.167	×	(1-0.10)	=	0.150	÷	0.767	= 0.196
Lung cancer	0.278	×	(1-0.30)	=	0.194	÷	0.767	= 0.254
							0.767	1.000

Hemoptysis-Fever								
Pulmonary tuberculosis	0.222	×	(1-0.70)	=	0.067	÷	0.717	= 0.093
Pulmonary embolism	0.333	×	(1-0.30)	=	0.233	÷	0.717	= 0.325
Brochiectasis	0.167	×	(1-0.00)	=	0.167	÷	0.717	= 0.233
Lung cancer	0.278	×	(1-0.10)	=	0.250	÷	0.717	= 0.349
							0.717	1.000

Dyspnea-Cavity								
Pulmonary tuberculosis	0.148	×	(1-0.60)	=	0.059	÷	0.774	= 0.077
Pulmonary embolism	0.370	×	(1-0.00)	=	0.370	÷	0.774	= 0.478
Brochiectasis	0.037	×	(1-0.10)	=	0.033	÷	0.774	= 0.043
Lung cancer	0.444	×	(1-0.30)	=	0.311	÷	0.774	= 0.402
							0.774	1.000

Dyspnea-Fever

Pulmonary tuberculosis	0.148	×	(1-0.70)	=	0.044	÷	0.741	=	0.060
Pulmonary embolism	0.370	×	(1-0.30)	=	0.259	÷	0.741	=	0.350
Bronchiectasis	0.037	×	(1-0.00)	=	0.037	÷	0.741	=	0.050
Lung cancer	0.444	×	(1-0.10)	=	0.400	÷	0.741	=	0.540
					0.741				1.000

Expectoration-Cavity

Pulmonary tuberculosis	0.417	×	(1-0.60)	=	0.167	÷	0.672	=	0.248
Pulmonary embolism	0.010	×	(1-0.00)	=	0.010	÷	0.672	=	0.016
Bronchiectasis	0.469	×	(1-0.10)	=	0.422	÷	0.672	=	0.628
Lung cancer	0.104	×	(1-0.30)	=	0.073	÷	0.672	=	0.109
					0.672				1.000

Expectoration-Fever

Pulmonary tuberculosis	0.417	×	(1-0.70)	=	0.125	÷	0.695	=	0.180
Pulmonary embolism	0.010	×	(1-0.30)	=	0.007	÷	0.695	=	0.010
Bronchiectasis	0.469	×	(1-0.00)	=	0.469	÷	0.695	=	0.675
Lung cancer	0.104	×	(1-0.10)	=	0.094	÷	0.695	=	0.135
					0.695				1.000

***Mycobacterium* TB -Cavity**

Pulmonary tuberculosis	1.000	×	(1-0.60)	=	0.400	÷	0.400	=	1.000
Pulmonary embolism	0.000	×	(1-0.00)	=	0.000	÷	0.400	=	0.000
Bronchiectasis	0.000	×	(1-0.10)	=	0.000	÷	0.400	=	0.000
Lung cancer	0.000	×	(1-0.30)	=	0.000	÷	0.400	=	0.000
					0.400				1.000

***Mycobacterium* TB -Fever**

Pulmonary tuberculosis	1.000	×	(1-0.70)	=	0.300	÷	0.300	=	1.000
Pulmonary embolism	0.000	×	(1-0.30)	=	0.000	÷	0.300	=	0.000
Bronchiectasis	0.000	×	(1-0.00)	=	0.000	÷	0.300	=	0.000
Lung cancer	0.000	×	(1-0.10)	=	0.000	÷	0.300	=	0.000
					0.300				1.000

Step 5. Calculate partial P that each clinical data pair confers to each diagnosis

To calculate the partial P that each clinical data pair confers to each diagnosis in the differential diagnosis list, equation 8 is applied to the PP value of the clinical datum present and the S of the clinical datum absent for each diagnosis (see clinical data pair tables above.)

Notice that throughout these iterations of equation 8, the entire denominator remains unchanged for each clinical data pair and table. However, the numerator does change with each iteration; it assumes the value of the denominator term corresponding to the diagnosis being processed.

Step 6. Create mini-max tables

Now, we must determine the *total probability* that the partial probabilities mentioned in step 3, 4 and 5 confer to each diagnosis in the differential diagnosis list. This is achieved by creating a *mini-max table* for each diagnosis (see below.)

The first column of each mini-max table lists each clinical datum present. The second column lists the PP value of each clinical datum present; its bottom cell repeats the greatest of these values, which is the total P of the diagnosis *before* clinical data absent are considered. The next several columns show the partial P values that each clinical data pair confers to the diagnosis; the number of these columns equals the number of clinical data absent. The heading of each column shows the clinical datum absent and its S for the diagnosis. Each partial P value is transferred from the clinical data pair table to the mini-max table cell where the clinical data present and absent converge. The bottom cell of each column repeats the greatest partial P value appearing in the column. The last column repeats the smallest value appearing in each row. The bottom cell of this column, which also is the last cell of the mini-max table, repeats the greatest value of the column; it equals the total P of the diagnosis, *after* clinical data absent have been considered.

Mini-max tables

Mini-max table for tuberculosis

TUBERCULOSIS	PP value = partial P before considering clinical data absent	Partial P with Cavity absent S = 0.6	Partial P with Fever absent S = 0.7	MINIMUM VALUE IN EACH ROW
Cough present	0.276	0.151	0.113	0.113
Hemoptysis present	0.222	0.116	0.093	0.093
Dyspnea present	0.148	0.077	0.060	0.060
Expectoration present	0.417	0.248	0.180	0.180
MTb present	1.000	1.000	*1.000*	1.000
MAXIMUM VALUE IN EACH COLUMN	1.000	1.000	1.000	**Total P = 1.000**

MTb, *Mycobacterium tuberculosis*. The total probability of **tuberculosis** at this diagnostic step is the maximum value (**1.000**) in the last column.

Mini-max table for pulmonary embolism

PULMONARY EMBOLISM	PP value = partial P before considering clinical data absent	Partial P with Cavity absent S = 0	Partial P with Fever absent S = 0.3	MINIMUM VALUE IN EACH ROW
Cough present	0.172	0.236	0.165	0.165
Hemoptysis present	0.333	0.435	0.325	0.325
Dyspnea present	0.370	0.478	*0.350*	0.350
Expectoration present	0.010	0.016	0.010	0.010
MTb present	0.000	0.000	0.000	0.000
MAXIMUM VALUE IN EACH COLUMN	0.370	0.478	0.350	**Total P = 0.350**

The total probability of **pulmonary embolism** at this diagnostic step is the maximum value (**0.350**) in the last column.

Mini-max table for bronchiectasis

BRONCHIECTASIS	PP value = partial P before considering clinical data absent	Partial P with Cavity absent S = 0.1	Partial P with Fever absent S = 0	MINIMUM VALUE IN EACH ROW
Cough present	0.310	0.382	0.425	0.310
Hemoptysis present	0.167	0.196	0.233	0.167
Dyspnea present	0.037	0.043	0.050	0.037
Expectoration present	*0.469*	*0.628*	0.675	0.469
MTb present	0.000	0.000	0.000	0.000
MAXIMUM VALUE IN EACH COLUMN	0.469	0.628	0.675	**Total P = 0.469**

The total probability of **bronchiectasis** at this diagnostic step is the maximum value (**0.469**) in the last column. Were the second column not included in the calculation, total P of this diagnosis would be 0.628; see property 4 B of mini-max procedure (explained later, page 51.)

Mini-max table for lung cancer

LUNG CANCER	PP value = partial P before considering clinical data absent	Partial P with Cavity absent S = 0.3	Partial P with Fever absent S = 0.1	MINIMUM VALUE IN EACH ROW
Cough present	0.241	0.231	0.297	0.231
Hemoptysis present	0.278	0.254	0.349	0.254
Dyspnea present	0.444	*0.402*	0.540	0.402
Expectoration present	0.104	0.109	0.135	0.104
MTb present	0.000	0.000	0.000	0.000
MAXIMUM VALUE IN EACH COLUMN	0.444	0.402	0.540	**Total P = 0.402**

The total probability of **lung cancer** at this diagnostic step is the maximum value (**0.402**) in the last column.

Step 7. Determine total P of a diagnosis

In the mini-max table, the last column lists the smallest values of each row; the greatest value in this last column, repeated in the last cell of the table, equals the total P of the diagnosis. Therefore, the algorithm determines the total P of a diagnosis based on partial P values; it involves the following concepts:

1. A clinical data pair comprises a clinical datum present and a clinical datum absent.

2. A specific clinical data pair, that we call *determining clinical data pair*, determines the total P of a specific diagnosis.

3. Applying Equation 8 to the PP value of the clinical datum present and the S of the clinical datum absent in the determining clinical data pair, yields a specific partial P that we call *determining partial P* because it determines and equals the total P of the specific diagnosis.

4. A *specific cell* for this *determining partial P* exists in the mini-max table of this specific diagnosis.

   - In this specific cell, the mentioned clinical datum present converges with the mentioned clinical datum absent.

   - In this specific cell, the value (italicized) of the determining partial P was transferred from its clinical data pair table to the corresponding mini-max table.

   - In this specific cell, the value of the determining partial P is at once the smallest in its row and the greatest in its column (see below.)

To find the clinical data pair (determining clinical data pair) responsible for the current total P of a diagnosis, we must backtrack the steps that led from that pair to the total P. Start at the last cell (total P) of the mini-max table and ascend (following the arrows) to any cell with the same value, then go left on that row until any cell with the same value (the determining partial P) is encountered. The clinical datum present and the clinical datum absent that converge to this cell comprise the requisite clinical data pair (determining clinical data pair); the respective PP value and S are shown in the mini-max table.

Example: In the mini-max table of Lung Cancer (page 48) the last cell shows the current total P (0.402) of this diagnosis. Following the arrows takes us to another cell with the italicized value 0.402, which is the determining partial P. To this cell converge PP value (0.444) of dyspnea present and S (0.3) of pulmonary cavity absent. The determining clinical data pair dyspnea-cavity is responsible for the current determining partial P and total P (0.402.)

Mini-max tables are not based on Bayes formula and therefore circumvent the problem of clinical data independence and disease incompatibility.

Alternative methods exist for determining the total P of a diagnosis:

- *Mini-max* alternative establishes the *maximum partial P* in the last column as the *total P of the diagnosis.*

- *Maxi-min* alternative establishes the *minimum partial P* value in the last row as the *total P of the diagnosis.*

In all cases thus far examined, these two alternatives have yielded identical total P values; but playing with bizarre fictitious sensitivity values, we fabricated an example where the mini-max and the maxi-min alternatives yielded different total P values. It can be demonstrated that with only two diagnoses in the differential diagnosis list, mini-max and maxi-min alternatives always yield an identical result; when more than two diagnoses are processed, different results may be obtained on rare occasions. This demonstration is beyond the scope of this publication. Searching for a general principle that can predict when the two probabilities will be equal, Tomás Feder found three pertinent rules:

1. If a row exists in which each cell contains the maximum value in the corresponding column.

2. If a column exists in which each cell contains the minimum value in the corresponding row.

3. If and only if a cell exists that at once contains the minimum value in its row and the maximum value in its column; this value (determining partial P) equals the value of the diagnosis total probability.

If only one rule is satisfied, total P is equal for both mini-max and maxi-min alternatives. Rule 1 and rule 2 are sufficient but not necessary; they are too strong and imply rule 3. Rule 3 is necessary and sufficient.

Unless experimentation with a prototype program proves otherwise, actual clinical cases almost always comply with rule 3, yielding the same total P with both alternatives. We ascribe this behavior to the typical proportion among sensitivities and the fact that the partial P values in the rows of the mini-max table present a monotone relation. The latter means that when in one row the partial P value increases or decreases from one cell to the next, in the other rows the changes occur in the same direction.

Were such monotone relation broken and were the mini-max and maxi-min alternatives to yield different results, a possibility could exist that a clinical datum *present* with a PP value *smaller* than the current greatest PP value of clinical data present could still *increase* the total P of the diagnosis. This would contradict the general definition of the P of diagnosis (equation 6, page 40.)

If monotony is broken, a determining partial P that is at the same time the greatest partial P of its column and the smallest partial P of its row may not exist. In this case, two different partial P will exist, one determining the total P of the diagnosis with the mini-max alternative and another determining the total P with the maxi-min alternative. Were an incidental clinical case to occur, where mini-max and maxi-min results differ, we would favor the first alternative. The last column of the mini-max table lists partial P values that remain from *clinical data present* after being reduced by clinical data absent, whereas the last row lists partial P values of *clinical data absent* after being increased by clinical data present. It seems more reasonable to equal total P to the greatest partial P of clinical data present (mini-max alternative) rather than to the smallest partial P of clinical data absent (maxi-min alternative.)

- Average of mini-max and maxi-min alternative results (if unequal) as the *total P of the diagnosis.*

- Nash equilibrium result as the *total P of the diagnosis*: The mini-max procedure can be seen as a two-player game of antagonist clinical data present versus clinical data absent, where a novel combination of Nash equilibrium and a modified Bayes formula find its application to medical diagnosis. In the mini-max table, a maximizing player chooses a row for a datum present and tries to maximize the resulting value, and a minimizing player chooses a column for a datum absent and tries to minimize the resulting value. The cell where the chosen row and column intersect shows the resulting value of equation 8 applied to the corresponding PP value and S. In the mini-max alternative, the maximizing player is first in choosing the row and then the minimizing player chooses the column. In the maxi-min alternative, the minimizing player is first in choosing the column and then the maximizing player chooses the row. In both cases, the second player, knowing the selection of the first, is able to counter it with the optimal strategy (this is a deterministic strategy called pure strategy). The strategy becomes uncertain if both players must choose their rows and columns simultaneously, because none of them knows the strategy chosen by the other. In such a situation the maximizing player may assign to the rows, probabilities adding to 1, and the minimizing player may assign to the columns, probabilities adding to 1 (this is a probabilistic strategy called mixed strategy.) If a row has assigned probability p and a column has assigned probability q, the *probability of the intersecting cell to be chosen* at random is $p \times q$, a value different from the *partial P*, result of equation 8 applied to the corresponding clinical data present and absent. Multiplying $p \times q \times$ partial P for each cell and adding the results for all cells in the mini-max table, yields the expected value of the chosen cell (in our case the total P of the diagnosis.) One can show that such a game always has a Nash equilibrium (P, Q), that is a choice of a set P of probabilities p for the set of rows and a set Q of probabilities q for the set of columns (as described above), so that when the maximizing player chooses P the resulting value is minimized by Q, and when the minimizing player chooses Q the resulting value is maximized by P. Nash equilibrium calculates the optimal strategy determining P ($p_1...p_n$) and Q ($q_1...q_n$). The Nash equilibrium (P, Q) yields a value always between mini-max and maxi-min results, but different from the average of both. When mini-max and maxi-min results are equal, which is the typical scenario, the game is strictly determined, and the expected value calculated with Nash equilibrium equals this result. Ideally, one should always determine total P of the diagnosis by computing the Nash equilibrium. However, determination of sets P and Q is mathematically complex and could invest a greater computing time, without offering a significant advantage over the simpler mini-max alternative, given the negligible or no difference between mini-max and maxi-min results (page 80.) We presented the Nash equilibrium alternative only for the theoretical interest of combining it with Bayes formula, in a mini-max environment and as a stimulus for computer researchers to find other applications where probabilistic accuracy is more critical.

Step 8. Update the differential diagnosis list

Next, we again sort all diagnoses in the differential diagnosis list, according to decreasing total P values:

Differential diagnosis list	Total P
Tuberculosis	1.000
Bronchiectasis	0.469
Lung cancer	0.402
Pulmonary embolism	0.350

Note that the total P values of the diagnoses have changed and are more widely dispersed, but they still do not satisfy, except for tuberculosis, our threshold requirements for confirming as final or ruling out each of the other diagnoses. Accordingly, additional clinical data must be investigated. Then the mini-max procedure must be iterated with each additional clinical datum, and the total P of all diagnoses recalculated, until requirements for conclusion of the diagnostic quest are satisfied (page 87.)

***

Properties of the mini-max procedure

1. Each additional clinical datum present generates a new *row* in an existing mini-max table.

2. Each additional clinical datum absent generates a new *column* in an existing mini-max table.

3. A mini-max table (in typical cases where mini-max and maxi-min results are equal) has only one determining partial P cell, the value of which (italicized in the table) is *the smallest of its row and the greatest of its column*. The clinical datum present and the clinical datum absent that converge to this cell constitute the determining clinical data pair that originated this determining partial P, which equals the *total P* of the diagnosis.

4. When an additional clinical datum *present* is processed with the mini-max procedure, the total P of the diagnosis may increase, depending on its PP value. Typically, when an additional clinical datum *absent* is processed with the mini-max procedure, the greater its S, the more it decreases the P of the diagnosis. However, exceptions to this rule result from the effect this S has on the partial P of the other diagnoses that share the clinical data pair table, and from the interaction of the resulting partial P values in the mini-max table. The total P of the diagnosis will either decrease, increase, or remain unchanged:

   A. *Total P decreases.* Let's concentrate on a clinical data pair table. For a specific diagnosis, the S value of the clinical datum absent is *inversely* related to *its* partial P and *directly* related to the partial P values of the *other* diagnoses. An additional clinical datum absent typically reduces the total P of a diagnosis if its S is greater than the S of the absent clinical datum in the *determining clinical data pair*, in turn responsible for the current *determining partial P* of the diagnosis. If this condition is fulfilled, this new partial P will be smaller than the current determining partial P and becomes the new determining partial P that equals total P in the mini-max table.

   B. *Total P increases.* The mini-max procedure is not intended to increase the total P of a diagnosis based on clinical data absent. Nevertheless, this occasionally occurs, but only when a *first* clinical datum absent is processed; because at this point only one clinical datum absent column is generated, smaller values do not exist in the rows. The greatest partial P value in this column becomes the determining partial P and if it exceeds the current total P, it will replace the latter. Any subsequent clinical datum absent that is processed—regardless of its S value and resulting partial P—can only decrease the total P, because only the smallest partial P in a row can become a determining partial P. If we do not want a first clinical datum absent to increase the current total P of a diagnosis, then the second column of the mini-max table must be included in the calculation. In this way, we avoid violating the general rule that a clinical datum absent must never increase the total P. However, it is questionable whether an occasional increase due to a clinical datum absent is illegitimate and should be disallowed.

51

An example is the mini-max table for bronchiectasis (page 48), where the total P of this diagnosis would have been 0.628 (italicized) instead of 0.469, were the second column not included in the calculation.

C. *Total P does not change,* when a clinical datum absent does not fulfil any of the conditions for decreasing or increasing total P. This occurs frequently; furthermore, the total P of a diagnosis is quite resistant to change, especially for diagnoses with a great total P. This is an important advantage of the mini-max procedure, because it precludes ruling out a confirmed diagnosis (strongly supported by clinical data present) by some relatively unimportant clinical datum absent (as seen in the example of tuberculosis, page 42.)

5. The order in which clinical data are processed is irrelevant; it will change only the relative position of the generated new row or column without affecting the total probability of the diagnosis. This commutative property is intuitive and consistent with physician's experience.

6. When an additional clinical datum present or absent is incorporated into a mini-max table, the previously calculated partial P values of the diagnosis in the table remain unchanged and need not be recalculated. Such P values are retained in case a need arises to determine which clinical datum pair generated a partial probability in a cell. The algorithm need remember the values in the last column only. Whenever an additional clinical datum is processed, new clinical data pairs are generated and new partial P values are calculated. The algorithm then compares these new partial P values with the existing partial P values in the last column and calculates the new total P of the diagnosis.

7. An interesting property of the mini-max procedure is revealed when the sum of the total P of all diagnoses in the differential diagnosis list is substantially greater than 1; it suggests that not all such diagnoses are competing, but that some represent concurrent diseases. The degree of support that a clinical datum gives to a diagnosis is directly proportional to its corresponding PP value. This value can be found in the clinical datum list associated with the diagnosis or in the second column of the mini-max table. If all clinical data predominantly support the same diagnosis, the remaining diagnoses tend to compete and the sum of the probabilities of all diagnoses in the differential diagnosis list is close to 1. When some clinical data predominantly favor one diagnosis and other clinical data predominantly favor another diagnosis, these diagnoses tend to be concurrent; the sum of their probabilities will be considerably greater than 1. Concurrent diagnoses are supported by different clinical data; accordingly, each concurrent diagnosis can by itself attain a probability up to 1. The greater the sum of the probabilities, the greater the number of concurrent diseases.

8. When a clinical datum present *with* a PP value that approaches or equals 1 strongly supports or confirms a diagnosis, a clinical datum absent—regardless of its S value—*cannot* reduce the great P that such a clinical datum present confers to the diagnosis. This property also is true for concurrent diagnoses with great probability in the differential diagnosis list. This important advantage precludes a confirmed diagnosis from being ruled out by a relatively unimportant clinical datum absent (see tuberculosis example on page 42.) However, the P of a diagnosis *without* a confirming clinical datum present *may* be reduced by the S of such a clinical datum absent. Retaining diagnoses with great P, while simultaneously ruling out diagnoses with a small P, enables concurrent diagnoses to be distinguished from competing diagnoses. The manner in which the algorithm processes concurrent diagnoses will be addressed later (page 81.)

9. Occasionally, when an additional clinical datum changes the total P value of a diagnosis in a differential diagnosis list, it may result in a significant opposite P change in one or more of the other

diagnoses. Should such results be accepted or disregarded? Acceptance of the P changes in the other diagnoses contradicts the rule that each clinical datum should be processed for its corresponding diagnosis only. Experimentation with a prototype diagnostic program perhaps will solve this dilemma. In any event, the greater the total P of any diagnosis, the more it resists change.

10. Each time an additional clinical datum becomes available, the entire mini-max procedure is iterated recalculating the total P values of the diagnoses, simultaneously processing all present and absent clinical data. However, unchanged values in mini-max table cells do not need to be recalculated (property 6.)

What happens when a diagnosis with a great P, based on a clinical datum present with a PP value = 1, is confronted with an additional clinical datum absent with an S = 1? Would the clinical datum present or the clinical datum absent win the rule in/rule out contest? In an actual case, this confrontation would be impossible to occur because S = 1 means that this clinical datum is always present, contradicting its absence. Furthermore, the mini-max procedure precludes the discredit of a diagnosis with a great total P by a clinical datum absent (property 8 of mini-max procedure.)

A situation similar to that in the previous paragraph occurs when a diagnosis is evident, but an important clinical datum that is expected to be present is erroneously absent or unobserved. For example a patient with polyuria, polydipsia, and strong family history of diabetes mellitus does not manifest the expected hyperglycemia due to a laboratory error. Diabetes insipidus, psychogenic excessive water ingestion, renal disease, and other causes for the mentioned clinical data have been ruled out. Perhaps a routine should be included in the algorithm that detects such contradictions and recommends verification of the discordant clinical datum.

VI. BEST COST-BENEFIT CLINICAL DATUM NEXT TO INVESTIGATE

The best cost-benefit clinical datum next to investigate for presence or absence in a patient is an important function that can substantially shorten and reduce the cost of a diagnostic quest by precluding investigation of futile clinical data. This has important socioeconomic implications, especially in this era of managed care, when insurance companies curtail tests and procedures, and when physicians are rated by their proficiency in ordering tests in general.

Computers are faster and more accurate than the human brain in selecting the most convenient clinical datum next to investigate for presence or absence at each diagnostic step.

Our algorithm recommends the best cost-benefit clinical datum next to investigate based on cost, PP value, and S. Essential rule:

An important function of a diagnostic algorithm is to inform at each diagnostic step, the most useful clinical datum next to investigate, considering cost versus benefit.

Because the term *best cost-benefit clinical datum next to investigate in a patient* is lengthy, we shorten it to **best cost-benefit clinical datum**.

The best cost-benefit clinical datum function enables us to predict which new clinical datum will most increase or decrease the total probability (P) of a diagnosis, reducing the number of clinical data required to achieve a final diagnosis.

A recommended best cost-benefit clinical datum can be evaluated—before actually accomplishing the corresponding test or procedure—by *virtually* considering it either present or absent, while observing how much it improves the diagnostic outcome.

Initial clinical data collection (page 33) was achieved during the history and physical examination. We accepted whatever clinical data were revealed, without considering their rule-in or rule-out power. Subsequent clinical data collection is more selective, because we have a differential diagnosis list and a better-structured diagnostic process that enables to apply statistical and probabilistic concepts, and choose the best cost-benefit clinical datum, based on cost, positive predictive value, and sensitivity.

To select a best cost-benefit clinical datum, several steps must be followed:

Step 1. Select clinical data not yet investigated in the patient

The algorithm examines *every* diagnosis in the differential diagnosis list and selects from its respective disease model all clinical data *not yet investigated.* These clinical data differ from those initially collected; they are expected to be numerous because each disease model will contribute many new clinical data. However, only clinical data of appropriate cost and either of great PP value or great S need be investigated for presence or absence.

Step 2. Organize clinical data not yet investigated according to cost category, diagnosis, PP value, and S

Clinical data not yet investigated are organized according to three hierarchical levels (Fig. 3, next page.)

The *first level* is **COST CATEGORIES**, comprising four categories: none, small, intermediate, and great (page 29.) The *second level* is **DIAGNOSES**, comprising all diagnoses in the differential diagnosis list, identically repeated in each cost category, in order of decreasing P value. The *third level* is **CLINICAL DATA**, comprising two lists that we call **PP VALUE LIST** and **S LIST** containing only those clinical data that have a cost similar to the corresponding cost category. Both lists contain the same clinical data, but ordered according to decreasing PP value and decreasing S value respectively, and consequently these clinical data are shown with different sequence in each list.

Step 3. Recommend a new clinical datum as best clinical datum assuming it present

The algorithm moves to the lowest as-yet-unprocessed COST category, selects the as-yet-unprocessed DIAGNOSIS with greatest P, and from the corresponding PP VALUE LIST, selects the as-yet-unprocessed clinical datum with the greatest PP value. This PP value then is compared to the PP value of the clinical datum present in the *current* determining clinical data pair. The value of the latter appears in the bottom cell of the second column of the mini-max table for this diagnosis, and equals the current P of the diagnosis *before* processing clinical data absent. New clinical data with equal or smaller PP value can be disregarded because—even if present—they will not change the current P of this diagnosis; the algorithm moves to Step 4. When the new clinical datum has a PP value that exceeds the current P of the diagnosis before considering clinical data absent (bottom cell of second column), the algorithm recommends it as best cost-benefit clinical datum. The user then verifies whether this clinical datum is absent or present. When this clinical datum is absent, it is disregarded, because if able to change the total P of the diagnosis, it will be detected by the S loop at the next Step 4, which processes clinical data assumed absent. When the recommended best cost-benefit clinical datum is present, the algorithm generates a new clinical datum list headed by this datum, and the partial P of the diagnosis *before* considering clinical data absent assumes the PP value of this new datum. To

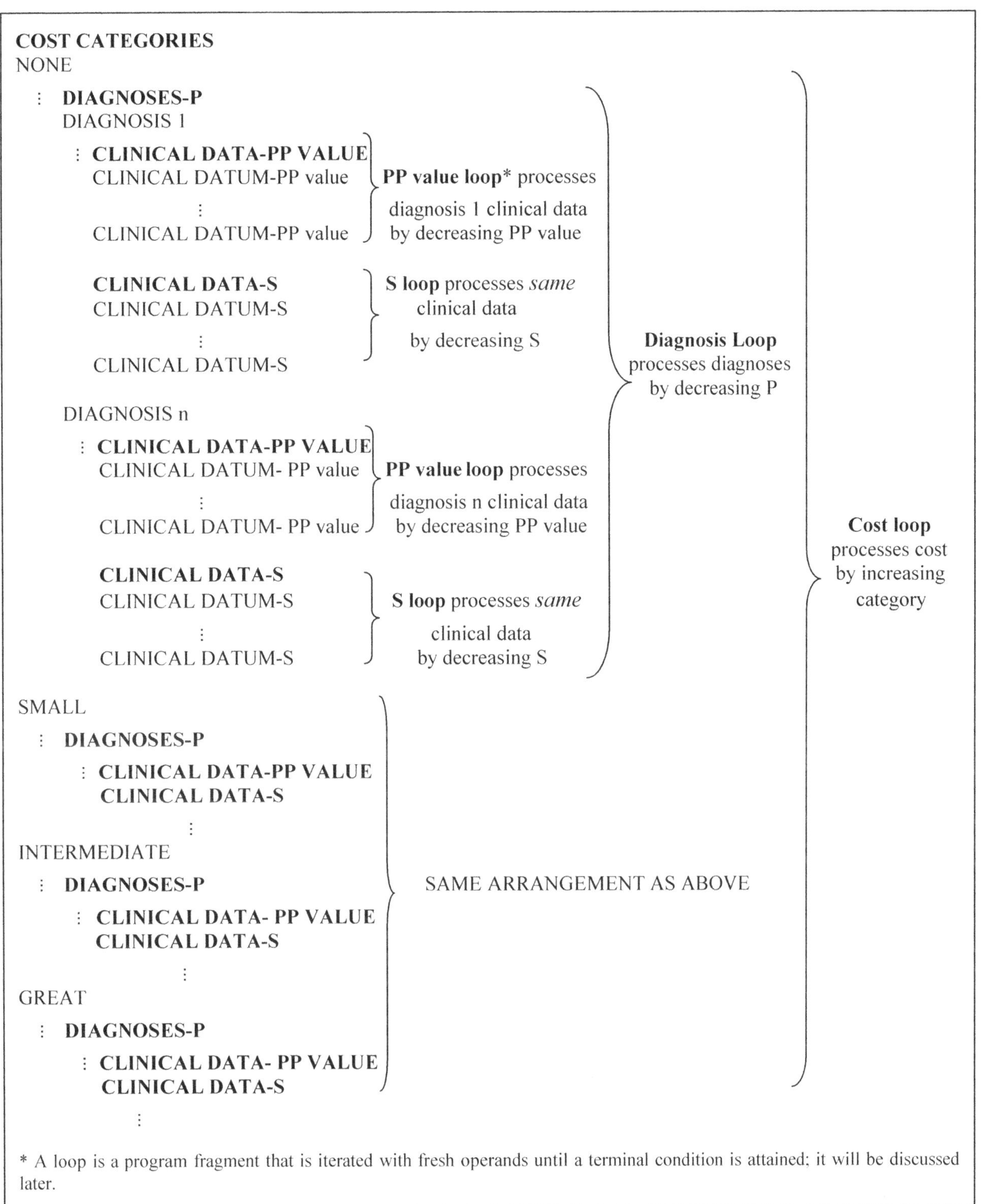

FIGURE 3. Nested loops for selecting best cost-benefit clinical datum.

recalculate the total P of the diagnosis *after* considering clinical data absent, several new clinical data pairs, combination of the best cost-benefit clinical datum present with each clinical datum absent, are generated; new clinical data pair tables are created and the partial P values for the diagnoses are calculated. A new row with these values is inserted in each mini-max table and the total P of the corresponding diagnoses are established.

Example: Assume we need to know whether the clinical datum pulmonary mass as evidenced by X-ray plain films, when *present*, can *increase* the current total P of lung cancer (see mini-max table for Lung Cancer on page 48.) The PP value of a pulmonary mass for lung cancer, stored in the disease model in the knowledge base, is 0.857. Equation 6 (page 40) states that the greatest PP value of the clinical data supporting a diagnosis equals the P value of this diagnosis:

$$P_{\text{lung cancer}} = \max (PP\ value_{\text{cough}},\ PP\ value_{\text{hemoptysis}},\ PP\ value_{\text{dyspnea}},\ PP\ value_{\text{expectoration}},\ PP\ value_{\text{MTb}},\ PP\ value_{\text{mass}})$$

$$= \max (0.241, 0.278, 0.444, 0.104, 0.000, 0.857) = 0.857$$

Accordingly, the previous P of lung cancer (0.444), *before considering clinical data absent* (bottom cell of second column in the lung cancer mini-max table), is increased to its new value of 0.857. The algorithm then creates a new clinical datum list:

Pulmonary mass	S	PP value
Lung cancer	0.9	0.857
Pulmonary tuberculosis	0.1	0.095
Pulmonary embolism	0.05	0.048
Bronchiectasis	0.0	0.000

To determine the total P of the diagnosis, *after considering clinical data absent*, the algorithm creates two new clinical data pair tables and calculates the partial P values for lung cancer:

Mass-Cavity	PP value	S		Partial P
Lung cancer	0.857	× (1-0.30) = 0.600	÷ 0.686	= **0.875**
Pulmonary tuberculosis	0.095	× (1-0.60) = 0.038		
Pulmonary embolism	0.048	× (1-0.00) = 0.048		
Bronchiectasis	0.000	× (1-0.10) = 0.000		
		0.686		

Mass-Fever	PP value	S		Partial P
Lung cancer	0.857	× (1-0.10) = 0.771	÷ 0.833	= **0.925**
Pulmonary tuberculosis	0.095	× (1-0.70) = 0.028		
Pulmonary embolism	0.048	× (1-0.30) = 0.034		
Bronchiectasis	0.000	× (1-0.00) = 0.000		
		0.833		

In the mini-max table for lung cancer, the algorithm creates a new row that shows these partial P values; then, the total P of this diagnosis *after* considering clinical data absent is calculated:

Mini-max table for lung cancer when pulmonary mass is present

LUNG CANCER	PP value = P before considering absent clinical data	Cavity absent S = 0.3	Fever absent S = 0.1	MINIMUM VALUE IN EACH ROW
Cough present	0.241	0.231	0.297	0.231
Hemoptysis present	0.278	0.254	0.349	0.254
Dyspnea present	0.444	0.402	0.540	0.402
Expectoration present	0.104	0.109	0.135	0.104
MTb present	0.000	0.000	0.000	0.000
Pulmonary mass present	0.857	*0.875*	0.925	0.857
MAXIMUM VALUE IN EACH COLUMN	0.857	0.875	0.925	**Total P = 0.857**

MTb, *Mycobacterium tuberculosis*

The total P of **lung cancer** at this diagnostic step is the maximum value (**0.857**) in the last column. Because of pulmonary mass *present* in chest X-ray plain films, the total P of lung cancer increased from 0.402 to 0.857.

Notice that except for the last two rows, partial P values shown in all other cells remain unchanged. However, the value and cell location of the determining partial P changed.

Each new best cost-benefit clinical datum present creates a new clinical datum list that includes the diagnosis from which it was selected. This diagnosis appears in some or all previous clinical datum lists because it originated the search for the new clinical datum; the latter just increases the number of clinical data that support this diagnosis and its P. Some of the new clinical datum lists may include previously unlisted diagnoses that also may manifest this clinical datum (Fig. 4.) When this occurs, such new diagnoses will not have clinical data in common with any previous diagnosis because they were not included in previous clinical datum lists; accordingly, previous and new diagnoses, if confirmed as final, must be concurrent. New clinical datum lists bring up new diagnoses; these, in turn, bring up new clinical data. At first thought, this cycle may seem to iterate indefinitely until the universe of clinical data is exhausted. In reality, this does not occur, because a single patient cannot manifest all clinical data. At some point, the newly recommended best cost-benefit clinical datum will simply be absent and will not create a new clinical datum list, aborting the cycle; still, it must be investigated so as to confirm its absence. Neither can a patient be afflicted by a multitude of concurrent diseases. Another factor limiting the number of diagnoses is that a best cost-benefit clinical datum is selected for its great PP value and accordingly is either pathognomonic for a single diagnosis or supportive of only a few diagnoses.

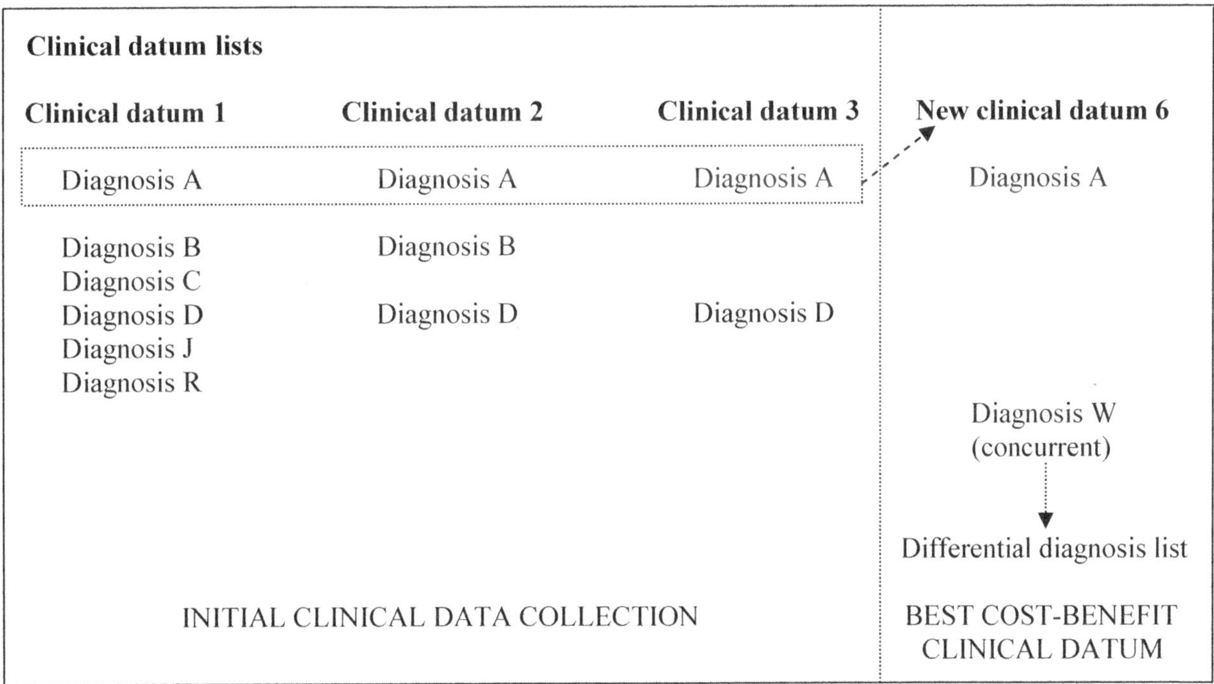

FIGURE 4. To increase probability of diagnosis A, supported by clinical data 1, 2, and 3 (dotted box), clinical datum 6 is recommended as best cost-benefit clinical datum. Clinical datum 6, confirmed present in the patient, creates clinical datum list 6 that includes diagnosis A from which PP list clinical datum 6 was selected; this increases P of diagnosis A and also the number of supporting clinical data. Previously unlisted diagnosis W, also supported by clinical datum 6, is included in the differential diagnosis list as a new diagnosis; if it reaches confirmation threshold, it will become a *concurrent* final diagnosis.

Step 4. Recommend a new clinical datum as best clinical datum assuming it absent

Typically, the greater the S of a clinical datum absent, the more it decreases the total P of a diagnosis. However, with the mini-max procedure, a clinical datum absent can occasionally increase total P (mini-max property 4 B, page 51) and it also can occur that a clinical datum with a smaller S can decrease total P more than *another* clinical datum absent with a greater S.

To verify whether a new clinical datum absent will indeed decrease the total P, the mini-max procedure needs not always be applied in its entirety; to save computer time (although this is unlikely to be critical, considering the great speed of today's computers), Tomás Feder devised the 3-Step method (see below). Should the first or second of these steps prove that a clinical datum does not decrease the total P, the following steps would be rendered unnecessary and the algorithm would move to the next diagnosis or cost category.

Besides shortening the processing time, the 3-Step method also determines whether *another* clinical datum absent with smaller S value is nevertheless able to reduce the total P of a diagnosis. This determination is accomplished by the first step only; when a clinical datum absent is thus proved not to reduce the P, neither will another datum of smaller S, and the algorithm can move to the next diagnosis. This is not true for the second and third step; even when these steps prove that the new clinical datum absent does not reduce P, the *next clinical datum with smaller S* must be processed with the first step, to determine whether this smaller S clinical datum can reduce P.

In the same COST category and DIAGNOSIS in which a new best cost-benefit clinical datum assumed present was processed involving PP value list, the algorithm moves now to the S LIST. From this list, the clinical datum of greatest S, not yet selected, is selected and substitutes the clinical datum absent in the *current* determining clinical data pair, creating a new clinical data pair.

3-Step method to determine whether a new clinical datum absent will decrease total P

Step 4.1

In the newly created clinical data pair, equation 7 (page 42) is applied to the PP value of clinical datum present and S of the new clinical datum from the S list, assumed absent. When the resulting P equals or exceeds the current *total P* of the diagnosis, neither *this* nor any *other* clinical datum in the same S list will decrease the total P; steps 4.2 and 4.3 can be skipped and the 3-Step method can advance to the next diagnosis. Conversely, when the resulting P is smaller, total P of diagnosis under consideration *might* decrease; the resulting P is stored. Proceed with step 4.2.

Computational time: step 4.1 (applying equation 7) involves only one subtraction and one multiplication.

Example: Assume we need to know whether the clinical datum pulmonary mass as evidenced by chest X-ray plain films, when *absent*, can *decrease* the current total P of lung cancer, which is 0.402, as shown in the last cell of the corresponding mini-max table (page 48.) The P of lung cancer *before* considering clinical data absent was 0.444 (equals greatest PP value in the second column, corresponding to dyspnea present); S of pulmonary mass on X-ray films for lung cancer is 0.9, as shown in the corresponding S list. Substituting these values in equation 7, we obtain:

$$P = PP \text{ value} \times (1 - S) = 0.444\,(1 - 0.9) = 0.044$$

This total P (0.044) is smaller than the prior total P of lung cancer (0.402); therefore, absence of mass in chest X-ray films *might* decrease this P. Proceed with step 4.2.

Step 4.2

A *clinical data pair table* is generated for the newly created clinical data pair of step 4.1; this table is headed by the clinical data pair and lists all the diagnoses in the differential diagnosis list. For each diagnosis, equation 7 is iterated, being applied to the corresponding PP value and S that the heading clinical data pair has for this diagnosis, to obtain the corresponding not yet normalized P (these P values do not sum 1.) Now equation 8 (page 42) is applied *only* to the diagnosis with the S list from which the clinical datum with greatest S was selected. The numerator of equation 8 is the non-normalized P of this diagnosis and the denominator is the sum of all non-normalized P values corresponding to the diagnoses in the clinical data pair table (this sum is smaller than 1). The value of the numerator of equation 8 was calculated in step 4.1; in the denominator, the clinical data pair for each term is the *same*, but with PP values and S values related to the respective diagnoses. The result of equation 8 is the normalized partial P of the mentioned diagnosis.

When the resulting partial P for the diagnosis under consideration equals or exceeds the current P, neither step 4.2 nor step 4.3 will decrease this total P. When this happens, disregard the clinical datum being processed and iterate the 3-Step method with the next greatest S clinical datum in the S list for the same diagnosis, until step 4.1 proves that no *other* clinical datum with a smaller S can decrease the total P. Then, advance the 3-Step method to the next diagnosis. Conversely, when the resulting partial P is smaller than the current total P, the clinical datum absent *might* decrease total P; the resulting P is stored. Proceed with step 4.3.

Only if the new clinical datum later is confirmed to be absent, will a new column be generated in the mini-max table. At step 4.2, *only one* cell—at the convergence of the clinical datum present and clinical datum absent—of this column (see example below) can show the result of equation 8. This cell shows the partial P that this clinical data pair confers to the diagnosis; all other cells of this column remain blank. Because equation 8 was applied to a clinical data pair with a greater S than the previous one, we know that the resulting partial P is the smallest in its row, but we do not know yet whether it also will be the greatest in its column and become the determining partial P.

Note: step 4.2 involves equation 8, the numerator of which is equivalent to equation 7 and the denominator of which always is equal or typically smaller than 1. Accordingly, the result of equation 8 (partial P of the diagnosis in step 4.2) will always be greater than its numerator (P of the diagnosis in step 4.1.) For this reason, it is unnecessary to proceed with step 4.2 when step 4.1 already yielded a P that equals or exceeds prior P.

Computational time: step 4.2 involves the application of equation 7 to *all diagnoses* in *only one clinical data pair table*, and equation 8 to *only one diagnosis* in this table. Computational time equals step 4.1 (equation 7) times the number of diagnoses (denominator of equation 8) plus the sum of the resulting terms (one sum for each diagnosis) plus the division of the numerator by the denominator.

Example (continued): create the dyspnea-mass clinical data pair table with the differential diagnoses showing the respective PP values and S values and then apply equation 7 to each diagnosis:

Dyspnea-Mass	PP value	S		
Pulmonary tuberculosis	0.148	$\times$	$(1-0.10)$	$= 0.133$
Pulmonary embolism	0.370	$\times$	$(1-0.05)$	$= 0.352$
Bronchiectasis	0.037	$\times$	$(1-0.00)$	$= 0.037$
Lung cancer	0.444	$\times$	$(1-0.90)$	$= 0.044$

Then apply equation 8 *only* to the diagnosis being processed, to obtain the partial P that this clinical data pair confers to this diagnosis:

$$P_{\text{lung cancer}} \;=\; \frac{\text{PP value}_{\text{lung cancer}}\,(1 - S_{\text{lung cancer}})}{\text{PP value}_{\text{lung cancer}}(1 - S_{\text{lung cancer}}) + \text{PP value}_{\text{TB}}(1 - S_{\text{TB}}) + \text{PP value}_{\text{embolism}}(1 - S_{\text{embolism}}) + \text{PP value}_{\text{bronchiectasis}}(1 - S_{\text{bronchiectasis}})}$$

$$P_{\text{lung cancer}} \;=\; \frac{0.444\,(1 - 0.90)}{0.444\,(1 - 0.90) + 0.148\,(1 - 0.10) + 0.370\,(1 - 0.05) + 0.037\,(1 - 0.00)}$$

$$=\; \frac{0.044}{0.044 + 0.133 + 0.352 + 0.037} \;=\; 0.078$$

Dyspnea-Mass	PP value	S		Partial P
Pulmonary tuberculosis	0.148	× (1- 0.10) = 0.133		
Pulmonary embolism	0.370	× (1- 0.05) = 0.352		
Bronchiectasis	0.037	× (1- 0.00) = 0.037		
Lung cancer	0.444	× (1- 0.90) = 0.044 ÷ 0.566	= 0.078	
		0.566		

We now can include in the mini-max table the new column "Mass absent", listing only one partial P conferred by the dyspnea-mass clinical data pair to lung cancer diagnosis; the other cells of the column remain empty.

Mini-max table for lung cancer when pulmonary mass is absent

LUNG CANCER	PP value = P before considering absent clinical data	Cavity absent S = 0.3	Fever absent S = 0.1	Mass absent S = 0.9	MINIMUM VALUE IN EACH ROW
Cough present	0.241	0.231	0.297		
Hemoptysis present	0.278	0.254	0.349		
Dyspnea present	0.444	0.402	0.540	0.078	0.078
Expectoration present	0.104	0.109	0.135		
MTb present	0.000	0.000	0.000		
MAXIMUM VALUE IN EACH COLUMN	0.444	0.402	0.540		

MTb, *Mycobacterium tuberculosis*

Because 0.078 is smaller than 0.402 (the current total P), the possibility remains that this total P *might* be decreased. Proceed with step 4.3.

Step 4.3

All possible new clinical data pairs and their tables are created, with each clinical datum present combined with the new clinical datum absent. In step 4.2, equation 7 was applied to all diagnoses in only one clinical data pair table, and then equation 8 was applied only to the diagnosis being processed, but now in step 4.3, equation 8 is applied to the same diagnosis in *all* the clinical data pair tables. This calculates the partial P values that the new clinical data pairs confer to this diagnosis; these partial P values show in *all* cells of the new column of the mini-max table (page 59.) This enables to determine the total P of the diagnosis, showing whether the absent clinical datum of greatest S indeed decreases it. If so, this clinical datum is recommended as the best cost-benefit clinical datum next to investigate; otherwise it is disregarded and the algorithm moves to the next diagnosis.

Computational time: equals the duration of step 4.2 multiplied by the number of new clinical data pairs.

Example (continued): create the remaining new clinical data pair tables and iterate equation 8 for lung cancer in all of them:

Dyspnea-Mass	**PP value**	**S**				**Partial P**
Pulmonary tuberculosis	0.148	×	(1- 0.10)	= 0.133		
Pulmonary embolism	0.370	×	(1- 0.05)	= 0.352		
Bronchiectasis	0.037	×	(1- 0.00)	= 0.037		
Lung cancer	0.444	×	(1- 0.90)	= 0.044	÷ 0.566	= 0.078
				0.566		

Cough-Mass						
Pulmonary tuberculosis	0.276	×	(1-0.10)	= 0.248		
Pulmonary embolism	0.172	×	(1-0.05)	= 0.164		
Bronchiectasis	0.310	×	(1-0.00)	= 0.310		
Lung cancer	0.241	×	(1-0.90)	= 0.024	÷ 0.747	= 0.032
				0.747		

Hemoptysis-Mass						
Pulmonary tuberculosis	0.222	×	(1-0.10)	= 0.200		
Pulmonary embolism	0.333	×	(1-0.05)	= 0.317		
Bronchiectasis	0.167	×	(1-0.00)	= 0.167		
Lung cancer	0.278	×	(1-0.90)	= 0.028	÷ 0.711	= 0.039
				0.711		

Expectoration-Mass						
Pulmonary tuberculosis	0.417	×	(1-0.10)	= 0.375		
Pulmonary embolism	0.010	×	(1-0.05)	= 0.010		
Bronchiectasis	0.469	×	(1-0.00)	= 0.469		
Lung cancer	0.104	×	(1-0.90)	= 0.010	÷ 0.864	= 0.012
				0.864		

***Mycobacterium* TB-Mass**						
Pulmonary tuberculosis	1.000	×	(1-0.10)	= 0.900		
Pulmonary embolism	0.000	×	(1-0.05)	= 0.000		
Bronchiectasis	0.000	×	(1-0.00)	= 0.000		
Lung cancer	0.000	×	(1-0.90)	= 0.000	÷ 0.900	= 0.000
				0.900		

We now can complete the new column "Mass absent" in the mini-max table for lung cancer:

Mini-max table for lung cancer when pulmonary mass is absent

LUNG CANCER	PP value = P before considering absent clinical data	Cavity absent S = 0.3	Fever absent S = 0.1	Mass absent S = 0.9	MINIMUM VALUE IN EACH ROW
Cough present	0.241	0.231	0.297	0.032	0.032
Hemoptysis present	0.278	0.254	0.349	0.039	0.039
Dyspnea present	0.444	0.402	0.540	*0.078* ◄······►	0.078 ▲
Expectoration present	0.104	0.109	0.135	0.012	0.012
MTb present	0.000	0.000	0.000	0.000	0.000
MAXIMUM VALUE IN EACH COLUMN	0.444	0.402	0.540	0.078	**Total P = 0.078**

MTb, *Mycobacterium tuberculosis*

Were a pulmonary mass *absent*, the previous total P of lung cancer indeed would be reduced from 0.402 to **0.078**.

A clinical datum absent with a smaller S occasionally is able to reduce total P more than another with a greater S. This mandates processing the clinical datum in the S list immediately below that with greatest S, because this clinical datum, if absent, might further reduce P. Accordingly, the 3-Step method is iterated with clinical data with progressively smaller S until step 4.1 no longer reduces P. Manually processed examples demonstrated that such reduction of total P occurs only occasionally and ceases after one or a few clinical data with smaller S are processed, and does not significantly prolong selection of the best cost-benefit clinical datum. This is because only clinical data with slightly smaller S can additionally reduce the total P.

***

So far, we explained how a best cost-benefit clinical datum assumed *absent* is selected and recommended. Now, this best cost-benefit clinical datum must be investigated for actual presence or absence in the patient. When this clinical datum is present, it is disregarded, because it neither can decrease the total P of the diagnosis (general rule) nor increase the total P (were it able to do so, it would have been detected by the PP value loop in step 3, page 54.) When this clinical datum is absent, it possibly could be masked by a drug or concurrent disease interaction. If this clinical datum absent is flagged with an interaction identifier, the algorithm must check for a drug or disease able to mask it; if confirmed, the clinical datum absent is disregarded and the user notified. If the clinical datum absent is not masked, the greatest partial P in the new column of the mini-max table becomes the new determining partial P, and the total P of the diagnosis decreases to this value.

In summary, to select the best cost-benefit clinical datum to investigate next, the algorithm loops at three nested levels (Figure 3, page 55): outer, intermediate, and inner. (1) The outer *cost loop* processes clinical data not yet investigated in order of increasing cost category: none, small, intermediate, and great. (2) Within each cost category, the intermediate *diagnosis loop* processes the diagnoses of the differential diagnosis list in order of decreasing P because those with greatest P values, are the best candidates for a final diagnosis, and can sooner conclude the diagnostic quest. (3) The inner *clinical data loop* comprises two sub-loops: the first begins at the top of the PP value list and terminates when no clinical datum exists with a PP value greater than the PP value of the determining clinical data pair. The second sub-loop processes, within the same level, the clinical data sorted by decreasing S, terminating when no clinical datum exists, able to change the P of the corresponding diagnosis.

All diagnoses in each cost category are similarly processed. The user is prompted each time the loop goes to a greater cost category. The remaining differential diagnoses with their P are displayed and the user is asked whether he wants to proceed in the greater cost category or prefers a deferred diagnosis, diagnosis by exclusion, or empirical treatment. The entire looping process terminates when all final diagnoses are obtained, the cost exceeds the benefit, or all the clinical data able to change P of diagnoses are processed. Clinical data that have the greatest PP value or the greatest S typically involve costly pathological investigations, such as biopsy or even autopsy. To request a biopsy or even an autopsy for a patient with tonsillitis would make little sense. This exaggeration emphasizes the importance of initially considering the cost of a clinical datum, before evaluating its PP value or S. However, in an emergency or when a patient's condition is deteriorating, investigation of confirmatory clinical data of great PP value takes priority over cost.

The recommended best cost-benefit clinical datum could be a common symptom quickly asked or immediately observed by the physician. Should obtaining a clinical datum require an involved test or procedure, the diagnostic process must be interrupted until the result becomes available. The "position of the game board", so to say, must be saved in the computer and opportunely retrieved to continue the

62

"game", because each new clinical datum, with its presence or absence in the patient, sets a new stage for the selection of the next best cost-benefit clinical datum. A disease is not a static process. If the clinical picture changes considerably prior to obtaining the diagnostic procedure result, a new diagnostic evaluation must be accomplished, sometimes from the beginning.

VII. SIMULTANEOUS RECOMMENDATION OF BEST COST-BENEFIT CLINICAL DATA

Few diagnostic computer programs recommend a single best cost-benefit clinical datum next to investigate; I know of none that simultaneously recommends a **set** of such data.

Recommending one best cost-benefit clinical data at a time is impractical; were the patient to require several tests, he would need to be contacted repeatedly for additional instructions. For this reason, physicians often *simultaneously* order a set of several analyses, tests, or procedures; this approach is critical for emergency cases, where there is no time to wait for sequential results. Essential rule:

To be practical for diagnosing actual cases, it is essential that a computerized diagnostic program be able to simultaneously recommend a *set* of best cost-benefit clinical data next to investigate.

A computer can emulate such human behavior by iterating the best cost-benefit clinical data function, first assuming each newly recommended best cost-benefit clinical datum as virtually present and then as virtually absent, while observing the effect that each iteration has on the P of each diagnosis. Such iteration can be represented by a trichotomy tree (Fig. 5, next page.)

Each tree represents a single diagnosis in the differential diagnosis list. Virtual branches represent best cost-benefit clinical data present or absent; nodes represent the P and cost of the diagnosis. Each node originates three new branches. Four cost level iterations are involved; accordingly, the total number of branches is $3^1 + 3^2 + 3^3 + 3^4 = 120$. Each top branch originating at a node assumes that the best cost-benefit clinical datum—selected from the PP value list—is present; accordingly, it increases P of the diagnosis and is depicted by an ascending arrow. Each middle branch assumes that *this* best cost-benefit clinical datum is absent; accordingly, it is disregarded, does not change P, and is depicted by a horizontal arrow. Each bottom branch assumes that the best cost-benefit clinical datum—selected from the S list—is absent; accordingly, it decreases P and is represented by a descending arrow. The same middle branch also assumes that this best cost-benefit clinical datum, selected from the S list, is present, disregarded, and does not change P. Additionally, this middle branch represents situations in which no best cost-benefit clinical datum was found in either the PP value list or S list; accordingly, it offers no best cost-benefit clinical data to investigate. This reduces the best cost-benefit clinical data to investigate to only two branches per node, the top (present) and the bottom (absent) branches; the middle branch is preserved however, because it takes us to a next node. In the entire tree, the number of best cost-benefit clinical data to investigate (branches) now is reduced to 80. This result multiplied by the number of diagnoses (trees) in the differential diagnosis list yields the total number of best cost-benefit clinical data to investigate, provided no best cost-benefit clinical data are shared with other trees (diagnoses.)

A clinical datum frequently is shared by diverse diagnoses. However, a best cost-benefit clinical datum selected from the PP value list has a great PP value; and when present, it is either very characteristic for only a few diagnoses or pathognomonic for only one diagnosis. Such clinical data are typically not shared with any other tree. When a best cost-benefit clinical datum is selected from the S list, because of its great S, and is absent, it might be shared by diverse diagnoses, for which this clinical datum occurs frequently.

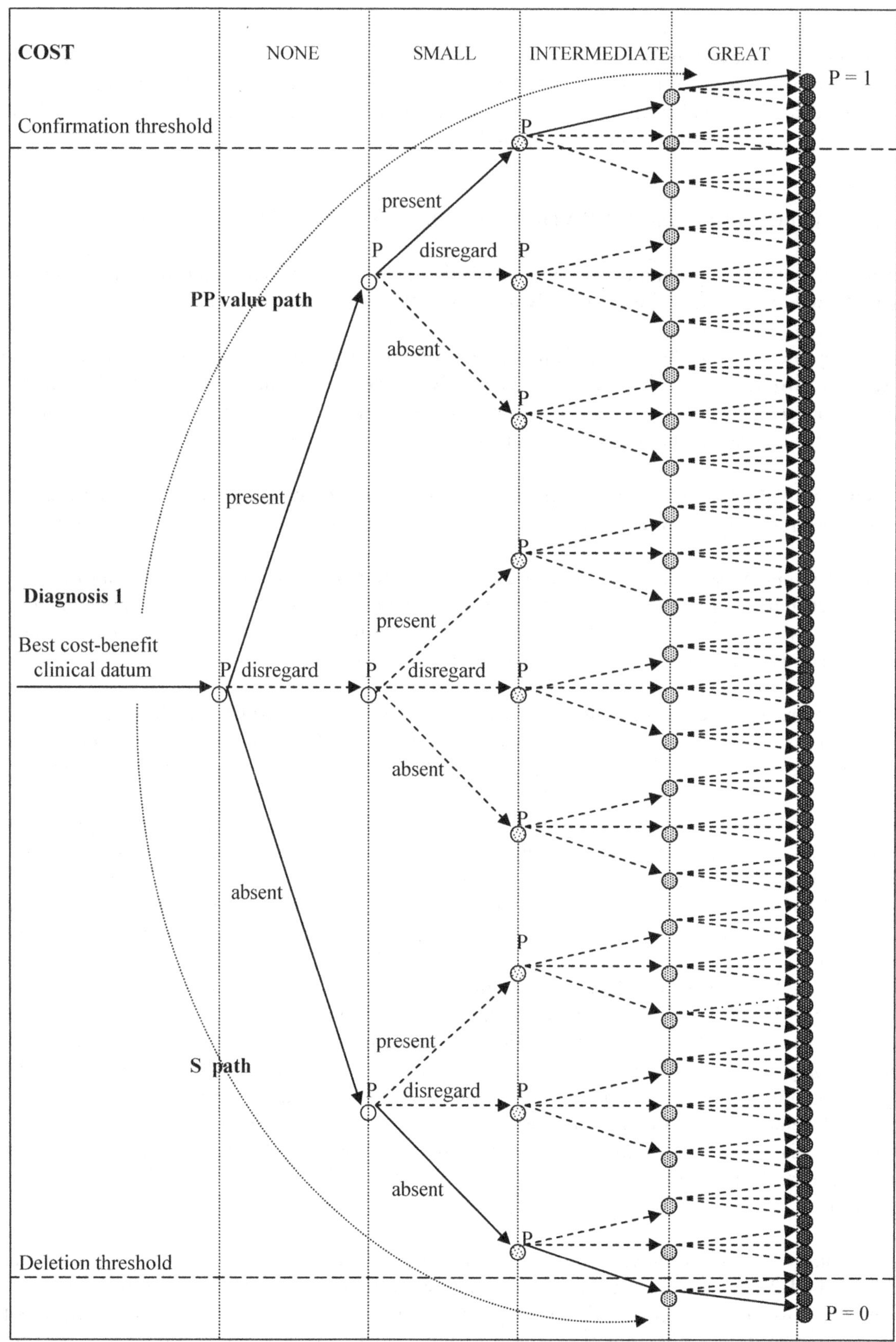

FIGURE 5. Trichotomy tree. Each branch (arrow) represents a best cost-benefit clinical datum. Each node (circle) represents the cumulative P and cost of the diagnosis.
○ NO COST; ◉ SMALL COST; ◍ INTERMEDIATE COST; ● GREAT COST

In a single tree, the best cost-benefit clinical datum present, represented by the top branch, typically has a great PP value and strongly supports a diagnosis. The best cost-benefit clinical datum absent, represented by the bottom branch, typically has a great S and strongly opposes a diagnosis. Occasionally, a best cost-benefit clinical datum, when it has a great PP value *and* a great S, may be recommended simultaneously in the top and bottom branch. This apparent opposition is not conflicting because it refers to *virtually present and absent alternatives* that do not coexist in a real patient case.

Processing the entire **set** of best cost-benefit clinical data perhaps could at once confirm as final those diagnoses with a P close to 1 and rule out those with a P close to 0. However, exhaustively traversing all branches of this exponentially growing trees is limited by the increasing number of clinical data to investigate and the cost involved. At best, the trichotomy tree approach may enable us to move only a few steps forward. Fortunately, heuristic shortcuts might dispel this concern. As noted on page 53, clinical data present of great PP value that strongly favor a diagnosis are unlikely to be opposed by clinical data absent of great S that strongly disfavor the same diagnosis. Accordingly, when a diagnosis with an initial great P is processed, we would expect the algorithm to recommend a best cost-benefit clinical datum of greater PP value that would further enhance that P, rather than recommend a best cost-benefit clinical datum of great S. Conversely, when a diagnosis with an initial small P is processed, we would expect the algorithm to recommend a best cost-benefit clinical datum of greater S that would further reduce that P, rather than recommend a best cost-benefit clinical datum of great PP value. This expectation would favor virtual traversing from present to present branches toward greater P values of the diagnosis or from absent to absent branches toward smaller P values of the diagnosis. Thus, in the tree of Fig. 5 the process would tend to traverse solid exterior branches only, while avoiding zigzag traversal along dashed alternating present and absent interior branches.

If we elect not to *exclusively* traverse extreme exterior branches, a few virtual best cost-benefit clinical data alternatively absent and present can be accepted. This maintains traversal *near* the exterior branches, leading to nodes with P near to diagnosis confirmation or elimination values.

Ideally, the algorithm explores—for each diagnosis in the differential diagnosis list—all possible virtual traversals until maximum or minimum P are attained, or until all available clinical data are exhausted. To accomplish this goal, prompts and authorization requests to continue in the next greater cost category must be bypassed. Cost momentarily is disregarded so as to obtain an ample overview of all best cost-benefit clinical data available. A decision regarding which best cost-benefit clinical data to select and up to what cost can be made afterwards according to disease severity and other circumstances.

NO COST clinical data are obtained as part of the initial consultation, from the history and physical examination. After evaluation of these NO COST clinical data, the user follows one or more of diverse strategies to select the most appropriate set of best cost-benefit clinical data next to investigate:

- Select *all* clinical data shown in the tree; this is possible only if the cost of acquiring them does not surpass an acceptable limit.

- Select only those clinical data of *lesser cost*. If, as a consequence, the diagnostic quest is not concluded, investigation of costlier clinical data can be pursued at a subsequent consultation. This strategy is consistent with standard medical practice.

- Select only best cost-benefit clinical data corresponding to *exterior branches* (represented by the solid arrows in Fig. 5) which traverse to a P that equals or approximates 1 or 0.

- Select preferably best cost-benefit clinical data *shared* by more than one diagnosis, when available; such data can be used for calculating P of more than one diagnosis.

Such selections can be made by the algorithm if parameters of cost, number of tests, and computational time limits can be provided.

The validity of the tree approach must be tested with a prototype computer program and actual patient cases.

***

VIII. DETAILED DISCUSSION OF MINI-MAX PROCEDURE

The example creating mini-max tables on pages 40 through 51 is didactic but oversimplified, because it assumed that each clinical datum list included a similar number of only four existing diagnoses. In reality, clinical datum lists include diverse number of diagnoses, from only one (when the clinical datum is exclusive—pathognomonic—for this diagnosis) to numerous (when the clinical datum, *e.g.*, fever, can be manifested by many diagnoses.) The all-inclusive method to integrate the differential diagnosis list (page 37) includes all diagnoses listed in all clinical datum lists (brought up by clinical data present). Consequently, the number of diagnoses in the differential diagnosis list will equal the number of diagnoses in the longest clinical datum list plus other diagnoses, not included in this longest clinical datum list, but listed in other clinical datum lists.

The number of diagnoses in the differential diagnosis list equals the number of terms in the denominator of equation 8 and the number of mini-max tables. New clinical data present or absent will add new rows or columns respectively to the existing mini-max tables. Only when a clinical datum present, creating a new clinical datum list, brings up a new diagnosis (see Fig. 4, page 57), such diagnosis is added to the differential diagnosis list, the corresponding term is added to the denominator of equation 8, and a corresponding new mini-max table is generated. This diagnosis, if confirmed final, will be concurrent to the previous ones because it does not share any of previously obtained clinical data; otherwise it would be listed in their clinical datum lists.

The diagnostic algorithm iterates from the start with each new clinical datum present or absent, and recalculates the probability of each diagnosis in the differential diagnosis list, including final confirmed diagnoses and deleted diagnoses. When it reaches the steps of creating clinical data pairs and clinical data pair tables (page 45), it automatically applies equation 8 to each clinical data pair and diagnosis, updating the denominator with all the terms, each corresponding to one of the diagnoses in the differential diagnosis list. When a term corresponds to a diagnosis that never manifests the clinical datum present in the clinical data pair, its PP value equals 0, and the entire term, PP value (1–S), equals 0 [0 (1–S) = 0] adding nothing to the denominator. When a term corresponds to a diagnosis that never manifests the clinical datum absent in the clinical data pair, its S equals 0, and the entire term, PP value (1–S), equals PP value [PP value (1–0) = PP value.] When a term corresponds to a diagnosis that never manifests the clinical datum present nor the clinical datum absent in the clinical data pair, its PP value and S equal 0, and the entire term, PP value (1–S), equals 0 [0 (1–0) = 0.] When a term corresponds to a diagnosis able to manifests both the clinical datum present and the clinical datum absent in the clinical data pair, the entire term equals PP value (1–S.)

So far, in the second *column* of each mini-max table, we listed PP values of clinical data present for the diagnosis considered; an alternative is to list, in this column, *partial P* that *clinical data present* confer to the diagnosis. To calculate these partial P, equation 8 is transformed by deleting all 1–S, which refer to clinical data absent, not pertinent at this point:

$$\text{Partial } P_i \text{ of diagnosis if clinical datum present} = \frac{\text{PP value}_i}{\text{PP value}_1 + \ldots + \text{PP value}_i + \ldots + \text{PP value}_n} \qquad (9)$$

Where: Partial P_i = partial P of diagnosis i under consideration, given a clinical datum present

PP value$_i$ = positive predictive value of clinical datum present being processed for diagnosis i

PP value$_1$…PP value$_i$…PP value$_n$ = positive predictive value of the same clinical datum present for each respective diagnosis in the differential diagnosis list

After initial clinical data collection and initial creation of mini-max tables, PP values equal these partial P values. This can be demonstrated by replacing each PP value in equation 9 with equation 5 and simplifying, in a similar way done on page 43, obtaining:

$$\text{Partial } P_i = \frac{S_i}{S_1 + \ldots + S_i + \ldots + S_n}$$

The right term of this equation is identical to the definition of PP value; therefore, partial P = PP value at this stage of the diagnostic process.

So far, in the first *row* of each mini-max table, we listed the names of clinical data absent with their respective S for the diagnosis considered; an alternative is to list *partial P* that *clinical data absent* confer to the diagnosis, listed in an added second row under the first. To calculate these partial P, equation 8 is transformed by deleting all PP values, which refer to clinical data present, not pertinent at this point:

$$\text{Partial } P_i \text{ of diagnosis if clinical datum absent} = \frac{(1-S_i)}{(1-S_1) + \ldots + (1-S_i) + \ldots + (1-S_n)} \qquad (10)$$

Where: Partial P_i = partial P of diagnosis i under consideration, given a clinical datum absent

S_i = sensitivity of clinical datum absent being processed for diagnosis i

S_1…S_i…S_n = S values of the same clinical datum absent for each respective diagnosis in the differential diagnosis list

P of a diagnosis given a clinical datum absent, is a concept closely related to negative predictive value.

Negative predictive value (NP value)

NP value is defined as conditional probability P of *disease absent* $\overline{D}$ given a clinical datum absent $\overline{C}$:

NP value = P $(\overline{D}|\overline{C})$

However, we need the partial probability of a *disease present* given a clinical datum absent: P $(D|\overline{C})$

NP value = P $(\overline{D}|\overline{C})$ = 1 – P $(D|\overline{C})$

P (D|C̄) = 1 – NP value

P (D|C̄) or 1 – NP value defines an index that represents the *strength with which a clinical datum absent disfavors a specific diagnosis* and equals partial P of a diagnosis given a clinical datum absent.

Although equations 5, 8, 9, and 10 derive from Bayes formula, they do not violate *independence* condition. PP value of a clinical datum present and S of a clinical datum absent, for each single diagnosis (in each single term of equation 8) or for unrelated diagnoses (diverse terms in denominator of mentioned equations) are independent. The mini-max procedure circumvents the *incompatibility* condition. The set of mini-max tables can be seen a three-dimensional deck, in which x-axis comprises clinical data absent, y-axis comprises clinical data present, and z-axis comprises the diverse mini-max tables (diverse diagnoses.) Such a set is cubic. Always remember that normalization is done in the direction of z-axis. Each cell of each table contains a partial P that is normalized and competes with partial P values of similarly located cells in all the other mini-max tables (summating 1), except cells in last column and last row, which contain respectively minimum and maximum partial P values. Conversely, partial P of cells in each *single* table are not normalized with partial P of other cells in this table; they are compared and minimums and maximums are computed in x- and y-axis directions respectively, determining total P of the corresponding diagnosis with this non-Bayesian procedure. *Exhaustiveness* is fulfilled as long as **all** diagnoses able to manifest a clinical datum are included in the denominator of the equations mentioned above.

Regarding exhaustiveness condition of Bayes formula, inclusion of "all diagnoses" can be interpreted in two manners:

(1) *All known diagnoses* (several thousands.) For equation 5 and 9, which process clinical data present, diagnoses unable to manifest a clinical datum (S = 0) will be represented by terms = 0 in the denominator; this addition of 0s to the denominator will not change its total value nor the result of the equation. For equation 10, which processes clinical data absent, diagnoses unable to manifest a clinical datum (S = 0) will be represented by terms 1 – S = 1 – 0 = 1). Adding such numerous 1s (several thousands) in the denominator would considerably reduce the resulting partial P.

(2) *All diagnoses potentially able to manifest a specific clinical datum* confirmed present (all those diagnoses that include this clinical datum in their disease models.) This clinical datum creates a clinical datum list; the less exclusive a clinical datum is, the more diagnoses will be listed in its clinical datum list, which could amount to a considerable number (*e.g.*, fever.) A diagnosis, to be included in the differential diagnosis list (ruled in), must be supported by at least one clinical datum present; in other words, a diagnosis must first be ruled in before it can be ruled out by clinical data absent (page 30.) Therefore, it makes sense to consider clinical data absent only for those diagnoses included in the differential diagnosis list, reducing the number of 1s to add in the denominator of equation 10 that calculates and normalizes partial P based on clinical data absent. Furthermore, the number of terms (diagnoses) in the denominator of equation 10 applied to diverse clinical data absent must be the same, to yield comparable values. To fulfill this condition it is necessary to look which clinical datum list includes the greatest number of diagnoses; then, the necessary 1 – 0 = 1 terms must be added to complete and equate this number for all calculations. This occurs automatically when the all-inclusive method to integrate the differential diagnosis list (page 37) is applied.

Effect of changes in the number of diagnoses in the differential diagnosis list on partial P values

Our all-inclusive method to integrate a differential diagnosis list (page 37) creates an initial list including all the diagnoses selected by the initially collected clinical data (page 33.) At this point, PP values equal partial P values of clinical data present. These values in the second column of the mini-max table are normalized (when they were calculated with equation 5), except the bottom cell, which shows the maximum value of the column (total P of diagnosis before clinical data absent are processed.) Because each diagnosis is represented by a term in the denominator of equations 8, 9, and 10, a change in the number of diagnoses in the differential diagnosis list produces a similar change in the number of these terms. This change affects the result of the mentioned equations: partial P values for clinical data present and partial P values for clinical data absent (1 − NP values), requiring recalculations involving re-normalizations. After re-normalization, PP values no longer equal partial P values for clinical data present; the total P of a diagnosis, before processing clinical data absent, equals now the greatest partial P of clinical data present (second column): total P = max (partial P_1...partial P_n.) Partial P for clinical data absent change, while S values do not. To preclude these changes, we maintain the number of diagnoses in the differential diagnosis list constant, by flagging confirmed final diagnoses and deleted diagnoses instead of removing them form this list.

Decrease in number of diagnoses (deletion or ruling out) in the differential diagnosis list reduces the number of terms in the denominator of equations 8, 9, and 10, increasing resulting partial P of remaining diagnoses. Occasionally, it might occur that a *new* clinical datum present strongly supports the deleted diagnosis (this relates to what was said on page 39, in the paragraph that mentions the "tip of the iceberg".) In this case the deleted diagnosis is recalled and its total P is recalculated and increased, reentering the competition with the remaining diagnoses, which partial P values decrease. The opposite situation of a confirmed final diagnosis, with great total P to be reduced by new absent clinical data is precluded by property 8 of mini-max procedure (page 52.) Retaining confirmed final diagnoses and deleted diagnoses in the differential diagnosis list (1) avoids the change in number of diagnoses and recalculation of partial P values; (2) enables occasional reprocessing of deleted diagnoses when a new clinical datum supports them more strongly than previous ones; (3) maintains the proper balance among P of competing diagnoses. Were a confirmed diagnosis, strongly supported by a clinical datum, removed from the differential diagnosis list, the next algorithm iteration might interpret that this clinical datum is exclusively supporting the remaining diagnoses and could confer them excessive P. A new clinical datum present may increase previous P of a diagnosis (because, selected from the PP value list, it has a greater PP value than the previous P); sometimes this clinical datum introduces also a new diagnosis, not listed in the previous clinical datum lists (Fig. 4, page 57.) Such new diagnosis will add a new term to the denominator of equation 8, and generate a new mini-max table. Because the new diagnosis was not listed in the previous clinical datum lists, it does not compete with previous diagnoses and will be concurrent. Although it ads a new term to the denominator of equation 8, this term equals 0 for all previous diagnoses; consequently, result of this equation remains *unchanged*, meaning that partial P in previous cells of mini-max tables do not need to be recalculated.

Axioms of our algorithm

1. S depends on a specific clinical datum and a specific diagnosis. Calculated with equation 2, page 24. The *greater* its value the stronger the clinical datum *absent* disfavors the diagnosis.

2. PP value depends on a specific clinical datum and a specific diagnosis. Calculated with equation 5, page 26. The *greater* its value the stronger the clinical datum *present* supports the diagnosis.

3. The greatest PP value of clinical data present supporting a diagnosis equals the P of this diagnosis before clinical data absent reduce this P. Calculated with equation 6, page 40.

S and PP values are fixed values that do not change with specific clinical cases; this enables pre-calculation of these values before the diagnostic program is applied to actual clinical cases, saving computing real time.

4. $P(D|\overline{C}) = 1 - NP$ value depends on a specific clinical datum and a specific diagnosis. The *smaller* its value the stronger the clinical datum *absent* disfavors the diagnosis. Calculated with equation 10, page 67. Pre-calculation of $1 - NP$ values for all clinical data and diagnoses, at an early stage when no diagnosis has been ruled in by a supporting clinical datum present and no differential diagnosis list has been created yet, is unpractical. As mentioned before (page 68), it would require to include thousands of 1s in the denominator, yielding very small $1 - NP$ values. The algorithm must calculate these values in real time, but now only for clinical data absent related to diagnoses supported by another clinical datum present and therefore included in the differential diagnosis list.

Calculation of PP values and S is necessary: (1) to process, with the mini-max procedure, initially collected clinical data. (2) To create PP value list and S list from which the best cost-benefit clinical datum next to investigate is selected to be compared respectively to PP values of clinical data present and S of clinical data absent in the existing determining clinical data pair; these values are compatible. If $1 - NP$ values are preferred in mini-max tables, a compatible so-called $1 - NP$ value list, similar to S list, cannot be pre-calculated, as mentioned above. Two solutions are envisioned: (a) a limited $1 - NP$ value list is calculated in real time, only for diagnoses in the differential diagnosis list, or (b) the S list can be utilized to select the top clinical datum with greatest S, and calculate only for this clinical datum the corresponding $1 - NP$ value, assuming that an equivalence between these two concepts exist, which is not always true (case of broken monotony, page 50.) PP values from the PP value list are equal and compatible with partial P for clinical data present (mini-max tables), as long as the number of diagnoses in the differential diagnosis list (number of terms in denominator) does not change. For this reason we do not remove from this list confirmed final diagnoses nor deleted diagnoses.

A tradeoff exists between the use of S and $1 - NP$ value of clinical data absent: S is more intuitive but requires the 3-Step method (page 58) to determine whether a clinical datum will indeed reduce P. $1 - NP$ value presents the mentioned difficulties to be calculated and is slightly less accurate than the 3-Step method. S values are already pre-calculated and available, whereas $1 - NP$ values must be calculated in real time. Each *mini-max table* requires only a $1 - NP$ value for each clinical datum absent; *$1 - NP$ value list* needs this value calculated for every diagnosis in the differential diagnosis list, to enable the selection of the clinical datum not yet investigated, with smallest $1 - NP$ value.

Summary of calculation of PP values and partial P values, and where they are applied:

$$\begin{array}{c} \text{Eq. 5} \qquad\qquad \text{Eq. 9} \\ S \longrightarrow \text{PP values} \longrightarrow \text{partial P of clinical data present} \\ \uparrow \qquad\qquad\qquad \uparrow \\ \text{PP value list} \qquad \text{mini-max table (second column)} \end{array}$$

$$\begin{array}{c} \qquad \text{Eq. 10} \\ S \longrightarrow 1 - NP \text{ values} = \text{partial P of clinical data absent} \\ \uparrow \qquad\quad \uparrow \qquad\qquad\qquad \uparrow \\ \text{S list} \qquad 1 - NP \text{ value list} \qquad \text{mini-max table (second row)} \end{array}$$

1 – S of clinical data absent, partial P of clinical data absent, and 1 – NP values are equivalent and interchangeable in all terms of equation 8. S of clinical data present, PP values, and partial P of clinical data present are also equivalent and interchangeable in equation 8 (as long as the number of diagnoses in the differential diagnosis list remain unchanged.)

If the use of partial P of clinical data absent or their equals 1 – NP values are preferable to 1 – S of clinical data absent, equation 8 becomes:

$$\text{Partial } P_i = \frac{PP\ value_i\,(1-NP\ value_i)}{PP\ value_1\,(1-NP\ value_1) + \ldots + PP\ value_i\,(1-NP\ value_i) + \ldots + PP\ value_n\,(1-NP\ value_n)}$$

Effect of new recommended best cost-benefit clinical data on partial P values

Recommended new best cost-benefit clinical data may create different situations, depending on whether selected from the PP value list or S list and whether present or absent in the patient.

If a new recommended best cost-benefit clinical datum selected from the PP value list is found absent, it is disregarded. If present, the new clinical datum creates a new clinical datum list that may comprise only the prior existing diagnosis from which PP list the new clinical datum was selected (*e.g.*, diagnosis A in clinical datum list 6, Fig. 4, page 57), increasing total P and number of clinical data that support this diagnosis. In this case, a new row for the new clinical datum present is added to all existing mini-max tables. At the next algorithm iteration, partial P values are calculated with equation 8, only for the new row, in each mini-max table; partial P values in second row (1 – NP values) do not change and do not need to be recalculated. When the new clinical datum list additionally includes a previously unlisted diagnosis (*e.g.*, diagnosis W in clinical datum list 6, Fig. 4), this new diagnosis creates a new mini-max table and adds a new row for the new clinical datum in the new and all previous mini-max tables. The new diagnosis changes partial P values for clinical data absent requiring also recalculation of second row with equation 10, in new and previous mini-max tables.

When the alternative of using a second row with 1 – NP values is preferred, the first cell of this row is shared with the second column (see example of comprehensive mini-max table, page 78.) This cell refers to the P of the diagnosis before clinical data present and absent are processed. As discussed on page 23, we disregard prevalence of disease, which gives each diagnosis equal prior probability. Consequently, this P is obtained dividing 1 by the number of diagnoses (n) in the differential diagnosis list. This result can be viewed also as obtained from equation 8 in which all PP values (of clinical data present) and all S (of clinical data absent) have been deleted.

$$P_i \qquad PP\ value_i\,(1-S_i)$$

If a newly recommended best cost-benefit clinical datum selected from the S list is found present, it is disregarded. If confirmed absent, it creates a kind of virtual clinical datum list, without the purpose to include its diagnoses in the differential diagnosis list, but only to obtain the respective S values, necessary to calculate the corresponding $1 - NP$ values with equation 10. A new column for the new clinical datum absent is added to all existing mini-max tables; no new table is generated because clinical data absent do not introduce new diagnoses. All partial P values of this new column are calculated, top cell with equation 10 and the other cells with equation 8. All previous partial P values in all tables remain unchanged.

For better visualization of the above statements, the following schematic mini-max tables and respective equations are presented in small print. Also refer to Fig. 4, page 57.

Old mini-max tables after adding clinical datum 6 present and diagnosis W

DIAGNOSIS A, B, C, D, J, or R	Clinical data absent →	Datum 4 $S \neq 1$	Datum 5 $S \neq 1$	MINIMUM VALUE IN EACH ROW
Clinical data present ↓	**Partial P of clinical data absent** → $1 \div (n+1) \neq 0$ [(1)] **Partial P of clinical data present** ↓	Eq. 10 $\neq 0$ [(2)]	Eq. 10 $\neq 0$ [(2)]	$\neq 0$
Datum 1 $S \neq 0$	Eq. 9 $\neq 0$ [(3)] unchanged	Eq. 8 $\neq 0$ [(4)] unchanged	Eq. 8 $\neq 0$ [(4)] unchanged	$\neq 0$ unchanged
Datum 2 $S \neq 0$	Eq. 9 $\neq 0$ [(3)] unchanged	Eq. 8 $\neq 0$ [(4)] unchanged	Eq. 8 $\neq 0$ [(4)] unchanged	$\neq 0$ unchanged
Datum 3 $S \neq 0$	Eq. 9 $\neq 0$ [(3)] unchanged	Eq. 8 $\neq 0$ [(4)] unchanged	Eq. 8 $\neq 0$ [(4)] unchanged	$\neq 0$ unchanged
New datum 6 **$S =$ or $\neq 0$** If $S = 0$ then all row $= 0$	**Eq. 9 $=$ or $\neq 0$** [(3)]	**Eq. 8 $=$ or $\neq 0$** [(4)]	**Eq. 8 $=$ or $\neq 0$** [(4)]	**$=$ or $\neq 0$**
MAXIMUM VALUE IN EACH COLUMN	$\neq 0$	$\neq 0$	$\neq 0$	**Total P $\neq 0$**

Unchanging maximum ⬚ ; Updated unchanging maximum ⬚ ; Column total maximum ⬚ (see text). "$=$ or $\neq 0$" in new clinical datum 6 line, means that if any of the previous diagnoses is included in its clinical datum list (such as diagnosis A in Fig. 4, page 57), result of equations 8 and 9 will be $\neq 0$; for any other diagnosis not included (meaning that clinical datum 6 is not a clinical datum of those diagnoses), result of equations 8 and 9 will $= 0$ in the corresponding mini-max tables.

[(1)] Eq. 11 (upper left cell):
$$\frac{1}{n + 1} \neq 0$$

n (number of diagnoses) is now one unit greater than before (added diagnosis W); consequently, partial P in upper left cell is smaller than before and has equal value in new and all old tables.

[(2)] Eq. 10 (second row):
$$1 - NP\ value_{A, B, C, D, J, R, or W} = \frac{1 - S_{A, B, C, D, J, R, or W}}{(1 - S_A) + (1 - S_B) + (1 - S_C) + (1 - S_D) + (1 - S_J) + (1 - S_R) + (1 - S_W)} \neq 0$$

Where: $S_{A, B, C, D, J, R, or W}$ = sensitivity of clinical datum absent for diagnoses A, B, C, D, J, R, or W.

1 – NP values (second row) are recalculated due to the addition of term $(1-S_W)$

$^{(3)}$ Eq. 9 (second column):

$$\text{Partial } P_{A,\,B,\,C,\,D,\,J,\,R,\,or\,W} = \frac{\text{PP value}_{A,\,B,\,C,\,D,\,J,\,R,\,or\,W}}{\text{PP value}_A + \text{PP value}_B + \text{PP value}_C + \text{PP value}_D + \text{PP value}_J + \text{PP value}_R + \text{PP value}_W} \neq 0$$

Where: PP value$_{A,\,B,\,C,\,D,\,J,\,R,\,or\,W}$ = PP value of clinical datum present for diagnoses A, B, C, D, J, R, or W.

Diagnosis W is not in the clinical datum lists 1, 2, nor 3, meaning that these clinical data are never manifested by diagnosis W: S_W and corresponding PP value$_W$ = 0. Consequently, the addition of new clinical datum 6, new diagnosis W, and corresponding new term 0 to the denominator, leaves equation 9 results (partial P for clinical data present) *unchanged* for old clinical data in old tables. But for clinical datum 6, S_W and PP value$_W \neq 0$, requiring calculation and normalization of partial P in the corresponding row, and recalculation of second row of all old and new tables.

$^{(4)}$ Eq. 8 (cells where clinical data present and clinical data absent converge):

$$\text{Partial } P\,(D|C_p \wedge C_a) = \frac{\text{PP value}_{A,\,B,\,C,\,D,\,J,\,R,\,or\,W}(1-S_{A,\,B,\,C,\,D,\,J,\,R,\,or\,W})}{\text{PPvalue}_A(1-S_A)+\text{PPvalue}_B(1-S_B)+\text{PPvalue}_C(1-S_C)+\text{PPvalue}_D(1-S_D)+\text{PPvalue}_J(1-S_J)+\text{PPvalue}_R(1-S_R)+\text{PPvalue}_W(1-S_W)}$$

Where: $P\,(D|C_p \wedge C_a)$ = partial P of diagnosis given a clinical datum present C_p *and* clinical datum absent C_a.

Diagnosis W is not in the clinical datum lists 1, 2, nor 3, meaning that these clinical data are never manifested by diagnosis W: PP value$_W$ = 0. Consequently, the addition of new clinical datum 6, new diagnosis W, and corresponding new term 0 to the denominator leaves equation 8 results *unchanged* for old clinical data in old tables. But for clinical datum 6, PP value$_W \neq 0$, requiring calculation and normalization of partial P of clinical datum 6 in the entire new row of all old and new tables, and recalculation of second row.

For programmers to save computing time, the following strategy is recommended: for each column compute the maximum value of all partial P for clinical data present (1, 2, and 3) and call it *unchanging maximum* (see mini-max table above.) Then, compute the maximum of this unchanging maximum and the partial P of new clinical datum 6 and call it *updated unchanging maximum*. Finally, compute the maximum of this updated unchanging maximum and the value in the top cell of the column (shared with second row) and call result *column total maximum*. With each new clinical datum investigated, the entire algorithm iterates from the start, but not all partial P values in the entire mini-max table need to be recalculated. Partial P of previous clinical data present do not change when a new clinical datum is introduced, as long as the number of diagnoses in the differential diagnosis list does not change; neither does the value of their maximum and for this reason we call it unchanging maximum. Conversely, the values in the second row of old mini-max tables change if a new diagnosis is introduced, and a new row with new partial P values is added by a new clinical datum present, requiring update of unchanging maximum and column total maximum. Consequently, only these changing values (second row, updated unchanging maximum, and column total maximum) need to be "remembered", be compared with the corresponding values calculated at the next algorithm iteration, and updated if appropriate. Because the algorithm adds only one new clinical datum at a time, at the start, the first clinical datum present entered in the mini-max table represents itself the first unchanging maximum, which will be updated at each next algorithm iteration.

New **mini-max table for diagnosis W after adding clinical datum 6 present**

DIAGNOSIS W	Clinical data absent $\rightarrow$	Datum 4 $S \neq 1$	Datum 5 $S \neq 1$	MINIMUM VALUE IN EACH ROW
Clinical data present $\downarrow$	**Partial P of clinical data absent** $\rightarrow$ $1 \div (n+1) \neq 0$ [(1)] **Partial P of clinical data present** $\downarrow$	Eq. $10 \neq 0$ [(2)]	Eq. $10 \neq 0$ [(2)]	$\neq 0$
Datum 1 $S = 0$	Eq. $9 = 0$ [(3)]	Eq. $8 = 0$ [(4)]	Eq. $8 = 0$ [(4)]	0
Datum 2 $S = 0$	Eq. $9 = 0$ [(3)]	Eq. $8 = 0$ [(4)]	Eq. $8 = 0$ [(4)]	0
Datum 3 $S = 0$	Eq. $9 = 0$ [(3)]	Eq. $8 = 0$ [(4)]	Eq. $8 = 0$ [(4)]	0
New datum 6 $S \neq 0$	**Eq. $9 \neq 0$** [(3)]	**Eq. $8 \neq 0$** [(4)]	**Eq. $8 \neq 0$** [(4)]	$\neq 0$
MAXIMUM VALUE IN EACH COLUMN	$\neq 0$	$\neq 0$	$\neq 0$	**Total P $\neq 0$**

[(1)] Eq. 11 (upper left cell):

$$\frac{1}{n+1} \neq 0$$

[(2)] Eq. 10 (second row):

$$1 - NP\ value = \frac{(1-S_W)}{(1-S_A) + (1-S_B) + (1-S_C) + (1-S_D) + (1-S_J) + (1-S_R) + (1-S_W)} \neq 0$$

[(3)] Eq. 9 (second column):

$$Partial\ P_W = \frac{PP\ value_W}{PP\ value_A + PP\ value_B + PP\ value_C + PP\ value_D + PP\ value_J + PP\ value_R + PP\ value_W}$$

Where: PP value$_{A, B, C, D, J, R,\ or\ W}$ = PP value of clinical datum present for diagnoses A, B, C, D, J, R, or W.

Diagnosis W is not in the clinical datum lists 1, 2, nor 3 meaning that these clinical data are never manifested by diagnosis W: $S_W = 0$. Consequently, the numerator and the entire equation $9 = 0$ for old clinical data in new table. New clinical datum 6 is manifested by diagnosis W; therefore PP value$_W \neq 0$ and equation $9 \neq 0$, requiring calculation and normalization of partial P of clinical datum 6 in corresponding row and recalculation and re-normalization of second column in all old and new tables.

[(4)] Eq. 8 (cells where clinical data present and clinical data absent converge):

$$Partial\ P\ (D|C_p{}^{\wedge} C_a) = \frac{PP\ value_W (1-S_W)}{PPvalue_A(1-S_A)+PPvalue_B(1-S_B)+PPvalue_C(1-S_C)+PPvalue_D(1-S_D)+PPvalue_J(1-S_J)+PPvalue_R(1-S_R)+PPvalue_W(1-S_W)}$$

Where: P $(D|C_p{}^{\wedge} C_a)$ = partial P of diagnosis given a clinical datum present C_p *and* clinical datum absent C_a.

Diagnosis W is not in the clinical datum lists 1, 2, nor 3 meaning that clinical data 1, 2, and 3 are never manifested by diagnosis W: $S_W = 0$. Consequently, the entire numerator and the entire equation 8 = 0 for old clinical data in new table. New clinical datum 6 is manifested by diagnosis W; therefore $S_{pW} \neq 0$ and equation $8 \neq 0$, requiring calculation and normalization of partial P of clinical datum 6 in corresponding row and recalculation and re-normalization of second column in all old and new tables.

Applying the described computing time saving strategy (page 73) to this case, unchanging maximum = 0; updated unchanging maximum = partial P in new row (datum 6); column total maximum = maximum of updated unchanging maximum and partial P in second row; because unchanging maximum = 0, remember column total maximum, second row, and updated unchanging maximum.

Mini-max tables after adding clinical datum 6 absent

DIAGNOSIS A, B, C, D, J, or R	Clinical data absent →	Datum 4 $S \neq 1$	Datum 5 $S \neq 1$	**New datum 6** $S \neq 1$	MINIMUM VALUE IN EACH ROW
Clinical data present ↓	**Partial P of clinical data absent →** $1 \div n \neq 0$ [1] unchanged **Partial P of clinical data present ↓**	Eq.10 $\neq 0$ [2] unchanged	Eq.10 $\neq 0$ [2] unchanged	**Eq. 10 $\neq 0$** [2]	$\neq 0$
Datum 1 $S \neq 0$	Eq. 9 $\neq 0$ [3] unchanged	Eq. 8 $\neq 0$ [4] unchanged	Eq. 8 $\neq 0$ [4] unchanged	**Eq. 8 $\neq 0$** [4]	$\neq 0$
Datum 2 $S \neq 0$	Eq. 9 $\neq 0$ [3] unchanged	Eq. 8 $\neq 0$ [4] unchanged	Eq. 8 $\neq 0$ [4] unchanged	**Eq. 8 $\neq 0$** [4]	$\neq 0$
Datum 3 $S \neq 0$	Eq. 9 $\neq 0$ [3] unchanged	Eq. 8 $\neq 0$ [4] unchanged	Eq. 8 $\neq 0$ [4] unchanged	**Eq. 8 $\neq 0$** [4]	$\neq 0$
MAXIMUM VALUE IN EACH COLUMN	$\neq 0$ unchanged	$\neq 0$ unchanged	$\neq 0$ unchanged	**$\neq 0$**	**Total P $\neq 0$**

[1] Eq. 11 (upper left cell):

$$\frac{1}{n} \neq 0$$

[2] Eq. 10 (second row):

$$1 - NP\ value = \frac{1 - S_{aA, B, C, D, J,\ or\ R}}{(1 - S_A) + (1 - S_B) + (1 - S_C) + (1 - S_D) + (1 - S_J) + (1 - S_R)} \neq 0$$

No new diagnoses; therefore no changes except for added new column for new clinical datum 6 absent; 1–NP value in second cell of this column is calculated and normalized. Of course, S_W is not included in denominator because new clinical data absent do not introduce new diagnoses.

[3] Eq. 9 (second column):

$$Partial\ P_{A, B, C, D, J,\ or\ R} = \frac{S_{A, B, C, D, J,\ or\ R}}{PP\ value_A + PP\ value_B + PP\ value_C + PP\ value_D + PP\ value_J + PP\ value_R} \neq 0$$

No new diagnoses; therefore, no changes in second column; of course S_W is not included in denominator.

[4] Eq. 8 (cells where clinical data present and clinical data absent converge):

$$P\ (D|C_p{}^{\wedge} C_a) = \frac{S_{pA, B, C, D, J,\ or\ R}\ (1 - S_{a\ A, B, C, D, J,\ or\ R})}{PPvalue_A(1 - S_A) + PPvalue_B(1 - S_B) + PPvalue_C(1 - S_C) + PPvalue_D(1 - S_D) + PPvalue_J(1 S_J) + PPvalue_R(1 S_R)}$$

No new diagnoses; therefore no changes except for added new column for new clinical datum 6 absent. All partial P in all previous cells remain unchanged; only all partial P values in new column are calculated and normalized. Of course S_W is not included in denominator.

Applying the described computing time saving strategy (page 73) to this case, all old cells remain unchanged; only the new column created by the new clinical datum absent adds partial P values. For each row (including second row) compute the minimum partial P and repeat it in a last column—only this column must be remembered.

How a new previously unlisted diagnosis can be introduced by a new best cost-benefit clinical datum was discussed above (Fig. 4, page 57.) Because the entire algorithm iterates from the start each time a new clinical datum is processed, the new diagnosis will automatically be added to the differential diagnosis list and processed with the mini-max procedure. One or more diagnoses also may be introduced by the *related clinical entities* routine (page 93-94.) When a diagnosis is introduced this way, previous clinical data do not support nor rule it in; otherwise it would already be listed in the respective clinical datum lists and differential diagnosis list. We add this diagnosis to the differential diagnosis list at Step 1 of best cost-benefit datum. This method will select all the clinical data listed in the corresponding disease model (because none was selected before), organize them by cost category, PP list and S list, and further process the diagnosis with the mini-max procedure, confirming it as final or ruling it out.

IX. SIMPLIFIED MINI-MAX PROCEDURE

Thus far, we have presented a comprehensive mini-max procedure, taking into account all the cells of the mini-max table. We also conceived an alternative simplified mini-max procedure, that is computationally shorter, faster, more efficient, although slightly less accurate.

The *comprehensive* procedure involves a mini-max table that is quadratic (number of rows *multiplied* by number of columns) because it includes all the cells to calculate total P of the corresponding diagnosis. It departs from the principle that the greater PP value of a clinical datum present the more P increases and the greater S of a clinical datum absent the more P decreases. However, with some clinical data absent, exceptions to the rule may occur (see property 4 of mini-max procedure, page 51) where a specific clinical datum absent can increase P instead of reducing it. The 3-Step method (page 58) must be applied to determine whether a clinical datum absent will indeed decrease total P, and whether some other clinical datum absent with smaller S than the previously processed can further decrease P. Although unlikely according to our tests, a possibility exists that the mini-max and the maxi-min alternatives do not yield equal total P (page 50.)

The *simplified* procedure involves a reduced mini-max table that is lineal (number of cells in second column *plus* number of cells in second row) because it disregards most of remaining cells. The table (depicted below, page 79) is integrated as follows:

First, P of the diagnosis before processing any clinical datum present and absent is calculated with equation 11 (page 71.) This value is located in the cell shared by the second column and second row, near the upper left corner of the table.

Second, partial P of clinical data present for each diagnosis in the respective mini-max table are calculated with equation 9 (page 67.) Partial P values are listed in the second column beside the corresponding names of clinical data present, listed in the first column.

Third, partial P values of clinical data absent for each diagnosis in the respective mini-max table are calculated with equation 10 (page 67.) These partial P values are listed in the second row below the corresponding names of clinical data absent, listed in the first row.

Fourth, equation 8 is applied only to the clinical datum present with greatest partial P (second column) and clinical data absent with smallest partial P or $1 - NP$ value (second row.) The resulting partial P is entered in the cell where greatest and smallest partial P values converge, and the total P is determined with the usual processing of minimum of rows and maximum of columns.

Example of a simplified mini-max table:

Only two clinical data present (clinical datum 1 and clinical datum 2), two clinical data absent (clinical datum 3 and clinical datum 4), and three diagnoses (diagnosis A, B, and C) in the differential diagnosis list are presented; only diagnosis A mini-max table is shown.

P of a diagnosis before processing clinical data present and absent (equation 11)

$$P = \frac{1}{\text{Number of diagnoses in the differential diagnosis list}} = \frac{1}{3} = \mathbf{0.333}$$

Clinical datum lists

Clinical datum 1, present	**S**	**PP value**
Diagnosis A	0.9	0.360
Diagnosis B	0.8	0.320
Diagnosis C	0.8	0.320

Clinical datum 3, absent	**S**	**PP value**
Diagnosis A	0.8	0.318
Diagnosis B	0.717	0.285
Diagnosis C	1	0.397

Clinical datum 2, present	**S**	**PP value**
Diagnosis A	0.2	0.414
Diagnosis B	0.283	0.586
Diagnosis C	0	0.000

Clinical datum 4, absent	**S**	**PP value**
Diagnosis A	0.1	0.091
Diagnosis B	0.5	0.455
Diagnosis C	0.5	0.455

Partial P conferred to the diagnosis by each clinical datum present (equation 9)

$$\text{Partial P conferred by clinical datum 1 to diagnosis A} = \frac{0.360}{0.360 + 0.320 + 0.320} = 0.360$$

$$\text{Partial P conferred by clinical datum 2 to diagnosis A} = \frac{0.414}{0.414 + 0.586 + 0.000} = 0.414$$

Partial P conferred by clinical datum 1 and 2 to diagnoses B and C are calculated similarly.

Partial P conferred to the diagnosis by each clinical datum absent (equation 10)

$$\text{Partial P conferred by clinical datum 3 to diagnosis A} = \frac{1-0.8}{(1-0.8)+(1-0.717)+(1-1)} = \frac{0.2}{0.2+0.283+0} = 0.414$$

$$\text{Partial P conferred by clinical datum 4 to diagnosis A} = \frac{1-0.1}{(1-0.1)+(1-0.5)+(1-0.5)} = \frac{0.9}{0.9+0.5+0.5} = 0.474$$

Partial P conferred by clinical datum 3 and 4 to diagnoses B and C are calculated similarly.

Partial P conferred to the diagnosis by each clinical data pair (equation 8)

Datum 1 – Datum 3   **PP value   S**   **P**
Diagnosis A $0.360 \times (1\text{-}0.8)$ $= 0.072$ (numerator) $\div 0.163$ (denominator) $= 0.443$
Diagnosis B $0.320 \times (1\text{-}0.717)$ $= 0.091$ (numerator) $\div 0.163$ (denominator) $= 0.557$
Diagnosis C $0.320 \times (1\text{-}1)$ $= \underline{0.000}$ (numerator) $\div 0.163$ (denominator) $= \underline{0.000}$
                                 Sum $= 0.163$ (denominator)   Sum $= 1.000$

Datum 1 – Datum 4   **PP value   S**   **P**
Diagnosis A $0.360 \times (1\text{-}0.1)$ $= 0.324$ (numerator) $\div 0.644$ (denominator) $= 0.503$
Diagnosis B $0.320 \times (1\text{-}0.5)$ $= 0.160$ (numerator) $\div 0.644$ (denominator) $= 0.248$
Diagnosis C $0.320 \times (1\text{-}0.5)$ $= \underline{0.160}$ (numerator) $\div 0.644$ (denominator) $= \underline{0.248}$
                                 Sum $= 0.644$ (denominator)   Sum $= 1.000$

Datum 2 – Datum 3   **PP value   S**   **P**
Diagnosis A $0.414 \times (1\text{-}0.8)$ $= 0.083$ (numerator) $\div 0.249$ (denominator) $= 0.333$
Diagnosis B $0.586 \times (1\text{-}0.717)$ $= 0.166$ (numerator) $\div 0.249$ (denominator) $= 0.667$
Diagnosis C $0.000 \times (1\text{-}1)$ $= \underline{0.000}$ (numerator) $\div 0.249$ (denominator) $= \underline{0.000}$
                                 Sum $= 0.249$ (denominator)   Sum $= 1.000$

Datum 2 – Datum 4   **PP value   S**   **P**
Diagnosis A $0.414 \times (1\text{-}0.1)$ $= 0.373$ (numerator) $\div 0.666$ (denominator) $= 0.560$
Diagnosis B $0.586 \times (1\text{-}0.5)$ $= 0.293$ (numerator) $\div 0.666$ (denominator) $= 0.440$
Diagnosis C $0.000 \times (1\text{-}0.5)$ $= \underline{0.000}$ (numerator) $\div 0.666$ (denominator) $= \underline{0.000}$
                                 Sum $= 0.666$ (denominator)   Sum $= 1.000$

Comprehensive mini-max table for diagnosis A

DIAGNOSIS A	**Clinical data absent →**	Datum 3 S = 0.8	Datum 4 S = 0.1	MINIMUM VALUE IN EACH ROW
Clinical data present ↓	**Partial P of clinical data absent →** 1 ÷ n = 0.333 **Partial P of clinical data present** ↓	0.414	0.474	0.333
Datum 1 S = 0.2	0.360	0.443	0.503	0.360
Datum 2 S = 0.1	0.414	0.333	0.560	0.333
MAXIMUM VALUE IN EACH COLUMN	0.414	0.443	0.560	MINI-MAX **Total P = 0.360** MAXI-MIN **Total P = 0.414**

The comprehensive mini-max procedure considers all cells (second column *multiplied* by second row). This example yields a total P of **0.360** with mini-max alternative and **0.414** with maxi-min alternative; a difference of 0.054. The S values have been selected to purposely produce broken monotony (page 50) and this difference in total P values for diagnosis A with mini-max and maxi-min alternatives; with real cases this situation seems to occur rarely if ever.

Simplified mini-max table for diagnosis A

DIAGNOSIS A	Clinical data absent →	Datum 3 S = 0.8	Datum 4 S = 0.1	MINIMUM VALUE IN EACH ROW
Clinical data present ↓	Partial P of clinical data absent → $1 \div n =$ *0.333 Partial P of clinical data present ↓	*0.414	0.474	0.333
Datum 1 S = 0.2	0.360			
Datum 2 S = 0.1	*0.414	*0.333		0.333
MAXIMUM VALUE IN EACH COLUMN	0.414	0.414		MINI-MAX Total P = 0.333 MAXI-MIN Total P = 0.414

The simplified procedure must calculate all the partial P in the second column—corresponding to clinical data present—to determine the greatest, and all the partial P in the second row—corresponding to clinical data absent—to determine the smallest. In this process the upper left cell is excluded because it does not represent any clinical datum. Once these greatest and smallest partial P are established, all other partial P (not emboldened) are disregarded. The mentioned greatest and smallest partial P, the partial P of the cell where they converge (calculated with equation 8 applied to the corresponding clinical data pair), and the now included upper left cell, define a 2 by 2 table (partial P flagged with asterisks.) Comparisons of values are done in the usual mini-max manner, obtaining 2 greatest values in last row and 2 smallest values in last column. The 4 values in the 2 by 2 table (flagged with asterisks) plus the 4 obtained values, plus the total P (lower right cell), all 9 embolden, configure a 3 by 3 table.

Schematic representation of a 3 by 3 table

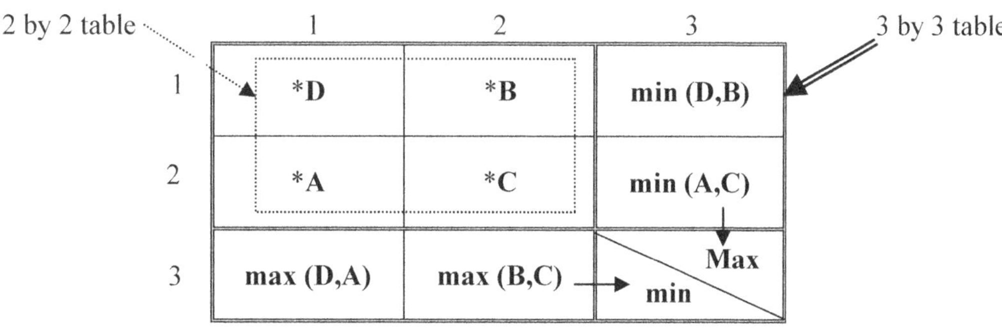

*A = greatest PP value or partial P of clinical data present (second column)

*B = smallest 1 – NP value or partial P of clinical data absent (second row)

*C = P (D|$C_p^\wedge C_a$) resulting from applying equation 8 to A and B

*D = $1 \div n$

Regardless of the size of the entire mini-max table, the total number of cells involved in determining the total P of the diagnosis equals the number of cells in the second column *plus* the number of cells in the second row *plus* the remaining 4 or 5 (if mini-max and maxi-min are unequal) cells necessary to complete the 3 by 3 table. Simplified mini-max procedure yields a total P of **0.333** with mini-max and **0.414** with maxi-min alternatives respectively; a difference of 0.081. Again, the S values for this example have been selected to purposely produce this difference in total P values for diagnosis A. The mentioned difference depends on the number of diagnoses in the differential diagnosis list; we established mathematically that it increases to a maximum of 0.15 with 9 diagnoses; with a greater number of diagnoses it starts gradually to decrease. Consequently, in this example, with the same clinical data we obtain three different total P values (0.360, 0.414, and 0.333), depending on which procedure and alternative we apply. As mentioned above, the greatest possible difference with the simplified mini-max procedure is 0.15, which appears insignificant for practical purposes and most likely will never occur.

In summary, the simplified mini-max procedure goes through the following steps:

1. Calculation of P of diagnoses before processing any clinical datum present and absent (upper left cell), dividing 1 by the number of diagnoses in the differential diagnosis list.

2. Calculation of partial P values, processing only clinical data present (second column) with equation 9.

3. Calculation of partial P values, processing only clinical data absent (second row) with equation 10.

4. Calculation of only one partial P value, processing clinical datum present with greatest partial P and clinical datum absent with smallest partial P with equation 8, for the cell necessary to complete the 2 by 2 and 3 by 3 tables.

5. Determination of total P of diagnosis by resolving the 3 by 3 table in the usual mini-max manner.

6. Iteration of steps 2, 3, 4, and 5 for each diagnosis in the differential diagnosis list.

The simplified mini-max procedure has two remarkable advantages:

1. Fewer partial P need to be calculated, because only one must be calculated with equation 8.

    Example: 10 clinical data present, 10 clinical data absent, and 10 diagnoses. With the comprehensive mini-max procedure, the number of partial P necessary to calculate is 10 (second column) $\times$ 10 (second row) $\times$ 10 (diagnoses) = 10^3 = 1,000. With the simplified mini-max procedure, the number of partial P necessary to calculate is only [10 (second column) + 10 (second row) + 1 (partial P of clinical data pair)] $\times$ 10 (diagnoses) = 210 partial P.

2. The quite cumbersome 3-step method (page 58) to verify whether a new clinical datum assumed absent will decrease the total P of a diagnosis, becomes unnecessary, because it is implicit in the simplified mini-max procedure. While the 3-Step method relies on S of the new clinical datum assumed absent, the simplified procedure relies on normalized partial P of clinical data assumed absent (equal 1 – NP value), calculated with equation 10.

    To verify whether a new clinical datum assumed absent will decrease the total P of a diagnosis, the simplified procedure checks whether its 1 – NP value is smaller than any of the values in the second row. If so, it adds its new column and equation 8 is applied to the *greatest* partial P in the second column and to the *smallest* partial P of the second row. The resulting partial P is included in the converging cell, completing the 2 by 2 table. Comparing these values in the usual mini-max manner generates the 3 by 3 table and determines whether this new clinical datum is able to decrease total P of diagnosis; if so it is recommended as best cost-benefit clinical datum next to investigate. After confirming that this clinical datum is indeed absent in the patient, it will decrease the total P; if present, it is disregarded. This procedure replaces first and second steps of the 3-Step method, which calculate only one partial P for the new column, disregarding the remaining partial P values in this column. Avoidance of the third step makes the simplified procedure somewhat less accurate, but this is compensated by its great advantages. Actually, if monotony is not broken, we know in advance that remaining partial P in new column will be smaller and therefore not necessary to be calculated. If monotony is broken, which rarely occurs if ever, then other cells in the column could be greater and mini-max result be unequal to maxi-min. We mentioned above that this inequality is minor and negligible.

Only for conceptual reasons, we mention an even shorter procedure that applies equation 8 to the greatest partial P of clinical data present (second column) and the smallest partial P of clinical data absent (second row); the result is directly considered the total P of the diagnosis. This procedure does not involve 2 by 2 table, 3 by 3 table, nor the usual determination of minimum and maximum values of rows and columns. Because the partial P values of second column and second row must be calculated anyway to find the respective greatest and smallest values, the processing time is not significantly reduced compared to the simplified procedure described above. For this reason and the greater inaccuracy involved, we do not endorse this short procedure.

Partial P needed to be remembered at each diagnostic iteration of mini-max procedure

To calculate new total P of diagnoses, which partial P values need to be remembered (registered) to be compared with corresponding values calculated at next algorithm iteration and updated? (1) For *comprehensive* mini-max procedure: the last column (mini-max alternative) if all-inclusive method to integrate a differential diagnosis list (page 37) is applied and its number of diagnoses remains unchanged. (2) For *simplified* procedure: the 2 by 2 table, which implies the 3 by 3 table, or the smallest partial P for clinical data absent, listed in second row, and the greatest partial P for clinical data present, listed in the second column. (3) For *short* procedure, only greatest partial P of clinical data present and smallest partial P of clinical data absent.

X. COMPETING AND CONCURRENT DIAGNOSES

Thus far, we have primarily concentrated on competing diagnoses in the differential diagnosis list, and the several probabilistic and heuristic methods for selecting the final diagnosis that corresponds to the patient's actual disease. Now, we will analyze several situations that may arise during the diagnostic process and relate them to the issue of competing diagnoses and concurrent diagnoses. We will illustrate these situations with clinical datum lists and Venn diagrams.

Situation I

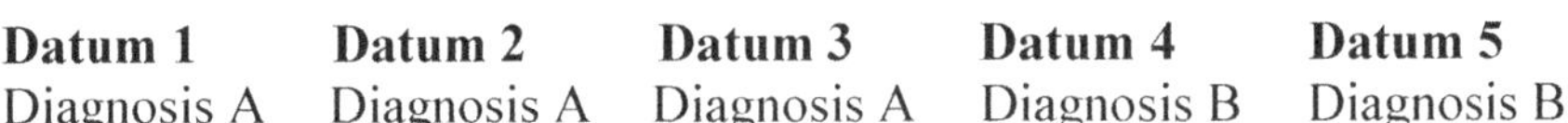

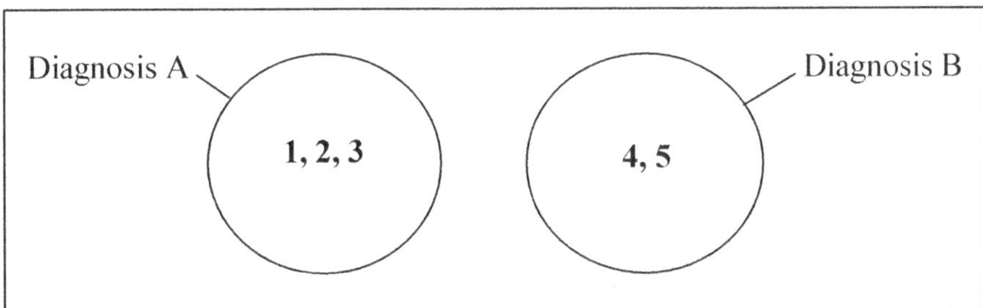

FIGURE 6. Venn diagram illustrating non-overlapping diagnoses A and B.

Diagnoses do not overlap (Fig. 6.) No single diagnosis accounts for all manifested clinical data. Diagnoses do not share clinical data.

Because all manifested clinical data must be rationalized—diagnosis A accounts for clinical data 1, 2, and 3, and diagnosis B accounts for clinical data 4 and 5—A and B clearly are concurrent diagnoses corresponding to concurrent diseases. Concurrent diagnoses can be independently processed in separate differential diagnosis lists, with the same algorithm used for a single disease; more than one final diagnosis will result. However, property 8 of the mini-max procedure (page 52) enables identification and separation of concurrent diagnoses in a single differential diagnosis list, superseding other more complicated methods.

Situation II

Datum 1	**Datum 2**	**Datum 3**
Diagnosis A	Diagnosis A	Diagnosis A
Diagnosis B	Diagnosis B	Diagnosis B

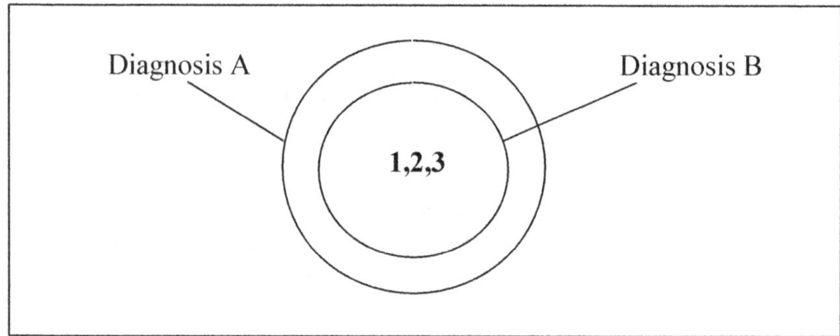

FIGURE 7. Venn diagram illustrating totally overlapping diagnoses A and B.

The diagnoses (two or more in some cases) totally overlap (Fig. 7.) More than one diagnoses account for all the manifested clinical data. All clinical data are shared by these diagnoses.

In this situation, A and B are likely competing diagnoses, because concurrent diseases rarely manifest identical symptoms. When the difference among the greatest P value (leading diagnosis) and the P values of the remaining diagnoses is small, additional clinical data, as recommended by the best cost-benefit clinical datum function, must be investigated for presence or absence, so as to increase the difference to a significant level. This may be at increased cost, if justifiable by the expected benefit.

Totally overlapping diagnoses can represent either concurrent diseases (unlikely) or competing diagnoses (likely); this likelihood typically resolves as new clinical data are obtained, resulting in Situation III. Should close P values of two or more diagnoses in the differential diagnosis list resist separation despite additional clinical data, concurrent diseases must be suspected. A clinical datum with great PP value for a diagnosis coexisting with another clinical datum with great PP value for another diagnosis reinforces the suspicion of concurrent diseases. When this occurs, the sum of the probabilities in the differential diagnosis list will be considerably greater than 1 (property 7 of the mini-max procedure, page 52.)

Situation III

The diagnoses partially overlap. Certain clinical data (overlapping region) are shared by the diagnoses; the remaining clinical data are unshared. This occurs in situation II, when additional clinical data are manifested in non-overlapping region.

1. When clinical data in a non-overlapping region belong to only one diagnosis, whether the overlapping diagnoses compete or are concurrent remains unclear because diagnosis A alone can account for all manifested clinical data (Fig. 8.)

Datum 1	**Datum 2**	**Datum 3**	**Datum 4**	**Datum 5**
Diagnosis A	Diagnosis A	Diagnosis A	Diagnosis A	Diagnosis A
Diagnosis B	Diagnosis B	Diagnosis B		

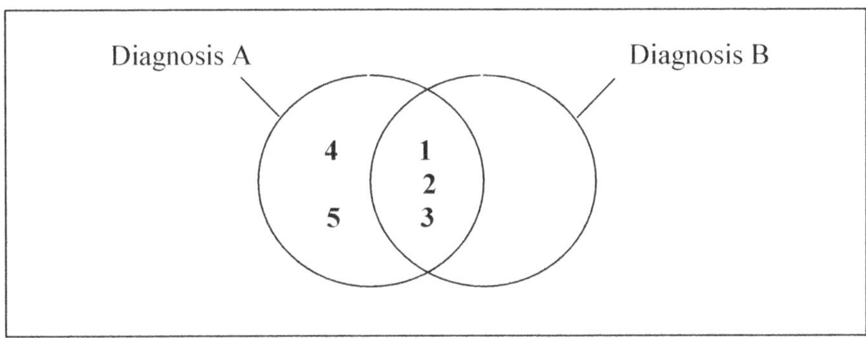

FIGURE 8. Venn diagram illustrating partially overlapping diagnoses A and B, with unshared clinical data (4, 5) in a single non-overlapping region.

Additional clinical data are required to clarify this situation. If additional clinical data are unavailable, the algorithm can proceed with the parsimony principle (page 38.) Diagnosis B will be considered competing and will be ignored if its P is small because it does not account for all clinical data, whereas diagnosis A does. However, the PP value of the clinical data in the overlapping region may tip the scale in one or the other direction. If the PP value of any of these shared clinical data is greater (more exclusive) for diagnosis A than B, then B is more likely to be a competing diagnosis. Conversely, if PP value is greater for diagnosis B than A, then diagnosis B is more likely to represent a concurrent disease. In other words, when the P of diagnosis A is greater than the P of diagnosis B, the latter is competing; when the P of diagnosis B is greater than A, the diagnoses may be concurrent. In the latter case the summed P values of all diagnoses in the differential diagnosis list will considerably exceed 1 (property 7 of mini-max procedure, page 52.)

2. When partially overlapping diagnoses include clinical data in more than one non-overlapping region, those clinical data belong to concurrent diagnoses. Diagnosis A accounts for clinical data 1, 2, 3, and 4; diagnosis B accounts for clinical data 1, 2, 3, and 5 (Fig. 9.)

Datum 1	**Datum 2**	**Datum 3**	**Datum 4**	**Datum 5**
Diagnosis A	Diagnosis A	Diagnosis A	Diagnosis A	
Diagnosis B	Diagnosis B	Diagnosis B		Diagnosis B

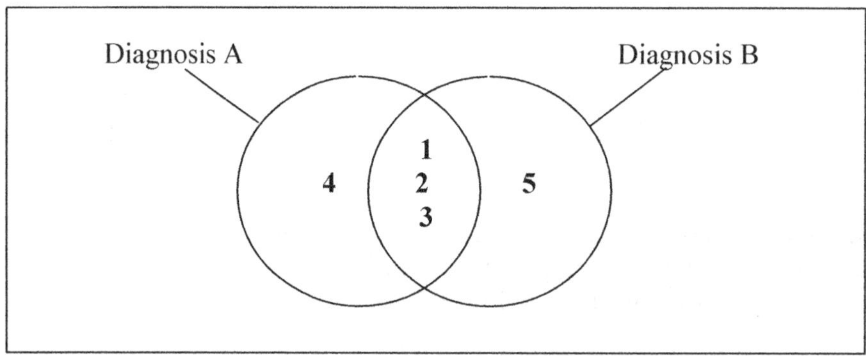

FIGURE 9. Venn diagram illustrating partially overlapping diagnoses A and B, with unshared clinical data (4, 5) in more than one non-overlapping region.

The clinical data in the overlapping region could mean that diagnoses A and B only coincidentally share these data, but otherwise are unrelated (see unrelated concurrence, page 93.) Alternatively, the shared data could mean a relationship between diagnoses A and B (see related concurrence, page 94) as in the example of metabolic syndrome, where insulin resistance is the shared clinical datum.

To confirm that diagnoses A and B are concurrent, the algorithm must search for unshared clinical data such as 4 and 5, each of which is exclusive to the respective disease model.

When the PP value of a shared clinical datum is greater for a specific diagnosis, that diagnosis probably accounts for this clinical datum. When the PP values of all shared clinical data are greater for one diagnosis, the other diagnoses compete; conversely, when some PP values are greater for one diagnosis and other PP values are greater for another diagnosis, those diagnoses are concurrent.

Another reason to suspect concurrence of diseases involves the mini-max procedure. Property 7 of the mini-max procedure (page 52) states: when the summed P values of all diagnoses in the differential diagnosis list substantially exceeds 1, some diagnoses are likely to be concurrent. The greater the sum, the more concurrent diseases exist.

Situation IV

Numerous overlapping diagnoses further complicate the diagnostic process.

Datum 1	Datum 2	Datum 3	Datum 4	Datum 5	Datum 6
Diagnosis A	Diagnosis A		Diagnosis A		
Diagnosis B		Diagnosis B	Diagnosis B	Diagnosis B	
			Diagnosis C		
		Diagnosis D		Diagnosis D	Diagnosis D

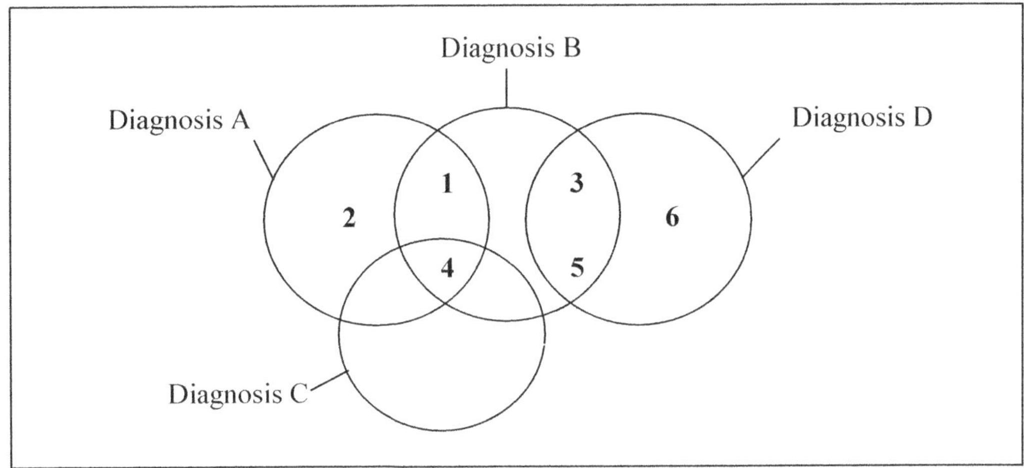

FIGURE 10. Venn diagram illustrating several partially overlapping diagnoses A, B, C, and D, with clinical data in overlapping and non-overlapping regions.

In this example, no single diagnosis can account for all manifested clinical data. No diagnosis is shared by all clinical datum lists; accordingly, some diagnoses must be concurrent. One diagnosis accounts for some clinical data; the remaining diagnoses account for the remaining clinical data. In this example (Fig. 10), four combinations of diagnoses account for all clinical data: (1) Diagnoses A, B, and D; (2) A and D; (3) A, C, and D; (4) A, B, C, and D. Diagnoses A and D clearly concur because they do not overlap. Diagnosis C either competes or concurs with either diagnosis A or diagnosis B in a manner similar to Situation III–1. Similarly, Diagnosis B can either compete or concur with combined diagnoses A and D; this latter combination alone also can account for all of the clinical data. A concurrent disease might have its own competing diagnoses.

Concurrent diagnoses raise several questions:

1. How does the algorithm *identify concurrent diagnoses*? Summarizing what was discussed earlier, some facts signal concurrence: (a) No overlapping of diagnoses (no sharing of clinical data) categorically confirms concurrence. (b) No single diagnosis will account for all manifested clinical data. (c) When concurrent diseases exist, more than one diagnosis with great P will remain atop of the differential diagnosis list. Processing additional clinical data will not increase—and may even decrease—differences among these probabilities. (d) The sum of probabilities of the diagnoses in the differential diagnosis list will be greater than 1—typically closer to 2 or more—depending on the number of concurrent diseases. (e) In case of overlapping diagnoses, some of the shared clinical data will stronger support one of the diagnoses (greater PP value for this diagnosis), while other clinical data will stronger support the other diagnosis (greater PP value for the other diagnosis.)

2. Which *combination of concurrent diagnoses* best accounts for all manifested clinical data, in case several possibilities exist (as described in above Situation IV and illustrated in Fig. 10)?

3. Is a *distinct differential diagnosis list* needed for each concurrent diagnosis and its competing diagnoses? The mini-max procedure seems to process well several concurrent diagnoses with a single differential diagnosis list. Because concurrent diseases may have their own competing diagnoses, some methods call for processing each concurrent disease in a distinct differential diagnosis list. When should the algorithm split the initial differential diagnosis list into such distinct differential diagnosis lists? One strategy would be to make such a split as soon as

concurrency is detected. If, from the beginning of the diagnostic process, we follow the comprehensive method of collecting as many clinical data as possible (see Initial Clinical Data Collection, page 33), we perhaps will have enough information to detect disease concurrence. But in general, this early ill-structured stage is inappropriate for discriminating concurrent diagnoses, especially when clinical data are collected using the abridged method. For this reason, an alternative strategy could be initially to combine all competing and concurrent emerging diagnoses in a single differential diagnosis list, splitting them into distinct differential diagnosis lists nearer the conclusion of the diagnostic process. At this stage, we have more clinical data, more diagnoses, and more accurate P values; the better structured diagnostic process facilitates choosing the most suitable method to select the best diagnostic combination able to account for all clinical data.

4. Can a single method simultaneously solve these problems?

Published algorithms offer only partial answers to these questions; some unanswered issues led me to devise my own solutions:

Mini-max method

Our algorithm relies on this method. Each diagnosis has its individual mini-max table. When strongly supporting clinical data are provided for each concurrent disease, the mini-max procedure maintains concurrent diagnoses (with great P) atop the differential diagnosis list. Such clinical data seem not to interfere much with the smaller P of other diagnoses. This suggests that all diagnoses with great P in the *single* differential diagnosis list are concurrent, whereas competing diagnoses are deleted. With other methods, concurrent diagnoses in a single differential diagnosis list are of concern because the algorithm may misinterpret them as competing diagnoses and, in an effort to eliminate all but one, recommends an inappropriately great number of clinical data. To preclude this futile loop, our preferred Double Threshold Method to Conclude the Diagnostic Quest (page 87) uses two empirical thresholds: an upper *confirmation threshold* and a lower *deletion threshold*. When a diagnosis reaches a confirmatory P value, it is flagged as final diagnosis. When two or more confirmed diagnoses are flagged in the differential diagnosis list and final diagnosis list, they correspond to concurrent diseases or concurrent clinical entities. This method of distinguishing concurrent from competing diagnoses supersedes more uncertain and cumbersome alternative methods; it satisfies all above questions.

Parsimony method

Looks for the diagnosis that either has the greatest P or accounts for the greatest number of clinical data and selects it as the first final diagnosis, then eliminates (?) the clinical data that this diagnosis rationalizes. Iterates the process for the remaining non-rationalized clinical data, and selects this second diagnosis as concurrent with the first. Iterates this process until all clinical data are rationalized. I have reservations concerning the elimination of clinical data rationalized by the first diagnosis before obtaining all concurrent final diagnoses. If the first diagnosis shares some clinical data with such concurrent diagnoses, removing such clinical data could reduce the chance of these concurrent diagnoses to become final. Therefore, an alternative would be to maintain all clinical datum lists until the diagnostic quest concludes. The parsimony method addresses questions 1 and 2, but whether it solves them accurately is unclear. Separate differential diagnosis lists are unnecessary.

Economy method

This method selects the smallest number of diagnoses that account for all clinical data, as exemplified by combination A and D in situation IV, Fig. 10. With this method, accuracy is uncertain; concurrent diagnoses must be identified by the methods summarized on page 85, question 1.

PP value method

When the PP value of clinical data in overlapping regions are greater for some diagnoses (conferring them greater probability) than for others, the combination that includes the former is favored (Page 83, situation III-1.) This method seems to be more accurate in identifying and combining concurrent diagnoses and possibly could function with a single differential diagnosis list. This method is embedded in our mini-max procedure that achieves it automatically.

XI. CONCLUSION OF DIAGNOSTIC QUEST

How does the human mind or the computer detect that the diagnostic process is completed and that a final diagnosis best represents the disease that afflict the patient? Several methods can determine when the conclusion of the diagnostic quest is achieved.

Double threshold method

Our algorithm is based on this method; it establishes two empiric thresholds: a *confirmation threshold* and a *deletion threshold*. When the P of a diagnosis in the differential diagnosis list is greater than the confirmation threshold, such diagnosis is flagged as *final*. When the P of a diagnosis in the differential diagnosis list is smaller than the deletion threshold, such diagnosis is flagged as *deleted*. The diagnostic quest concludes when all diagnoses in the differential diagnosis list are flagged. Flagging and maintaining final and deleted diagnoses in the differential diagnosis list, as opposed to removing them, keeps the number of diagnoses, the number of terms in the denominator of equations, and number of mini-max tables unchanged, avoiding recalculations of partial P values (page 69.) This method, based on the mini-max procedure, enables a *single* differential diagnosis list to comprise all concurrent, flagged final diagnoses, instead of a separate list for each, remarkably simplifying the identification and separation of concurrent from competing diagnoses. Final diagnoses are copied into a *final diagnoses list* and displayed together with the clinical data that support them.

Each concurrent final diagnosis requires a "clinching" clinical datum present (with PP value close to 1); very sensitive (S close to 1) clinical data absent rule out diagnoses. For final diagnoses, P = 1; for deleted diagnoses, P = 0. In actual practice, such extreme values are not required; the confirmation and deletion threshold values must be empirically determined.

Difference method

The greater the difference among the P of the leading diagnosis (that with the greatest P) and the P of the remaining diagnoses, the more likely the leading diagnosis will be final. The diagnostic process concludes when the P difference among the leading and remaining diagnoses exceeds an empirically established value.

Deletion method

Establishes an empiric P threshold below which a diagnosis is unlikely to become the final diagnosis; accordingly, every diagnosis with a P value below this threshold is deleted from the differential diagnosis list. The diagnostic process concludes when only the final diagnosis remains in the differential diagnosis list.

Difference and deletion methods require a separate differential diagnosis list for each concurrent disease.

Threshold values in all methods must be empirically established and stored in the knowledge base; they should be adjustable according to the severity of patient's condition, favorable or unfavorable evolution, prognosis, and availability of efficient treatments. This problem can be related to a type of *Receiver Operating Characteristic (ROC) curve* that tunes the diagnostic process. Decreasing a confirmation threshold may erroneously confirm a diagnosis of a disease that does not afflict the patient; increasing it precludes this error, but may require costlier clinical data to increase the P of the diagnosis to the level of this threshold. Increasing a deletion threshold may erroneously rule out a diagnosis of a disease that afflicts the patient; decreasing it precludes this error, but may require costlier clinical data to decrease the P of the diagnosis, to the level of this threshold.

XII. DISEASE AND DRUG INTERACTIONS

Drugs often interact, one enhancing or reducing the effects of another. Drugs also may adversely alter clinical data of a disease. In a somewhat similar manner, concurrent diseases may interact, one enhancing or reducing (*masking*) a clinical datum of another. Components of a clinical presentation (clinical entities) also can interact. Let's consider some examples:

- Chest pain of acute myocardial infarction may be masked by a concurrent diabetes or advanced age.

- A positive tuberculin reaction may be rendered negative by a concurrent immunosuppressive disease (AIDS) or a drug (*e.g.*, a corticosteroid.)

- A systolic hypertension may be reduced by concurrent acute myocardial infarction or shock.

- Inflammatory symptoms of rheumatic diseases or appendicitis may be suppressed by corticosteroids or antibiotics.

Disease and drug interactions are dangerous, because they can mask important clinical data and result in misdiagnosis. This is especially important in the diagnosis of life threatening diseases. Essential rule:

An efficient computer program must detect interactions among diseases and drugs.

The affected clinical datum in general is diminished in intensity or completely masked, as in the above examples; we are dealing with a clinical datum absent that would otherwise be present in the disease. In our diagnostic algorithm, the absence of an expected clinical datum tends to rule out the disease in direct proportion to the S of the datum. In the first example, chest pain in acute myocardial infarction has a great S (occurs very frequently.) With the mini-max procedure, absence of chest pain, a consequence of concurrent diabetic neuropathy, would greatly reduce the P of myocardial infarction and could have dismal consequences. Accordingly, if a concurrent disease cancels a clinical datum of the primary disease, S of this clinical datum must be proportionally reduced, to reduce its rule-out power. A practical solution is to reduce S of chest pain for myocardial infarction to zero in a diabetic patient; this is equivalent to eliminate chest pain from diagnostic consideration. In this case the diagnosis of myocardial infarction must be achieved with other clinical data present such as an ECG and cardiac enzymes.

Only certain specific clinical data of specific diseases are susceptible to be masked by concurrent diseases or drugs. We flag with interaction identifiers such clinical data in the corresponding disease models and list the potential masking diseases and drugs.

When a clinical datum absent of great S is processed, the algorithm checks whether it is flagged with an interaction identifier. Potentially interacting diagnoses are added to the differential diagnosis list to be confirmed or ruled out. The user is asked whether the patient is receiving specific drugs capable of interaction. When such an interacting diagnosis or drug is confirmed, S of the masked clinical datum is reduced to zero and the user alerted.

When a clinical datum assumed absent is found present, it is disregarded and no new column is generated in mini-max tables. When a clinical datum is confirmed absent but potentially masked by a concurrent disease or drug, it is also disregarded (S for the processed diagnosis reduced to 0), but a new column should be generated in all mini-max tables because the same clinical datum may not be masked in other diagnoses.

XIII. SAFETY CHECKS

A shortcoming of some computer diagnostic programs is the possibility of missing a diagnosis because of failure to collect adequate clinical data or to omit including the correct diagnosis in the differential diagnosis list. Four safety checks to minimize these errors are mentioned:

1. The algorithm checks for *interaction identifier* flagged clinical data, and proceeds as explained in the previous section.

2. The algorithm checks for *risk identifier* flagged *clinical data*. When a clinical datum *present* is risk flagged, the algorithm ensures that all diagnoses in the corresponding clinical datum list are included in the differential diagnosis list. This check is superfluous if the preferred all-inclusive method (page 37) is implemented, because it routinely includes in the differential diagnosis list all diagnoses of all clinical datum lists. When a clinical datum *absent* is risk flagged, it can be disregarded unless also interaction flagged, in which case it must be established whether indeed absent or masked.

3. The algorithm checks for *risk identifier* flagged *diagnoses*. If a diagnosis is risk flagged in a non-flagged clinical datum list, the algorithm must ensure its inclusion in the differential diagnosis list. Same as with the previous safeguard routine, this check is superfluous if the preferred all-inclusive method is implemented.

4. Once a final diagnosis is achieved, the algorithm searches the *complex clinical presentation models* (page 92) for links to possible causes, evolutionary stage, complications, etc.; if a match is established, the linked clinical entities of the model are included in the differential diagnosis list to be processed for presence or absence.

XIV. DIAGNOSES RELATED TO PATIENT SEX AND OTHER ATTRIBUTES

A diagnostic problem that arises is how the algorithm precludes diagnoses that exclusively afflict one sex—such as prostate diseases in men and ovarian diseases in women—from appearing in the differential diagnosis list of the opposite sex. A practical solution is to provide the knowledge base with a list of diagnoses that never can afflict a patient with a given sex, an have the algorithm preclude any of these diagnoses from being included in the differential diagnosis list. With our algorithm this blocking occurs automatically because sex is considered a clinical datum and could be included in each disease model with the corresponding PP value and S. Each male-exclusive disease model includes a "male sex" clinical datum that has $S = 1$ because it is always present in males, whereas PP value is very small (it is poorly characteristic) because many diseases afflict men. Likewise, each female-exclusive disease model includes a "female sex" clinical datum with $S = 1$ and very small PP value.

When a male-exclusive disease (*e.g.*, prostate cancer) is included in the differential diagnosis list of a female patient (*e.g.*, because of blood in urine), the algorithm will recommend "male sex" clinical datum as the best cost-benefit clinical datum because it has the greatest $S = 1$ in the S list. When this clinical datum is noted absent in the female patient, the mini-max procedure will reduce the P of the diagnosis to zero and the disease will be eliminated from the differential diagnosis list. A similar process occurs when a female-exclusive disease (*e.g.*, ovarian cyst) is included in the differential diagnosis list of a male patient. However, a method like this would be very inefficient because it would create a clinical datum list "female sex" or "male sex" including thousands of potential diagnoses, then transferred to the differential diagnosis list by the all-inclusive method (page 37), and each improper diagnosis would need to be ruled out one by one. We discussed the procedure anyway, as an example of how the mini-max procedure is able, although inefficiently, to delete these diagnoses based on great S of clinical data absent, and also because it could be applied to other attributes with shorter clinical datum lists, such as age, race, occupation, and others.

XV. DIAGNOSIS OF SOMATIZATION AND MALINGERING

Somatization and malingering typically yield many inconsistent clinical data and clinical datum lists, but no diagnosis is repeated in a majority of such lists. Convergence to a specific disease, syndrome, or clinical entity does not occur. The distancing of P values of diagnoses in the differential diagnosis list, typically experienced with physical diseases, does not occur. Objective clinical data investigated by physical examination are absent; tests and procedures yield normal results, which will rule out any physical disease.

XVI. EMPIRICAL TREATMENT

If two or more diagnoses remain not flagged as final or deleted in the differential diagnosis list, all of which are likely to respond to a single treatment, an empiric treatment may be warranted. If such treatment is successful, a more accurate but costlier final diagnosis will be unnecessary. For example, when only a few rheumatic diagnoses remain unflagged in the differential diagnosis list, empiric treatment with corticosteroids may be justifiable.

XVII. DEFERRED DIAGNOSIS

Therapeutic decisions often can be briefly deferred (Szolovitz and Pauker [16]) when achieving a final diagnosis would be costly and competing diagnoses are not immediately serious. Meanwhile, the patient may manifest clarifying clinical data or his disease may spontaneously resolve. The best cost-benefit clinical datum function facilitates the decision to defer diagnosis by alerting the user when the cost category increments.

Example 1: A patient presents with recent-onset fever; history and physical examination are otherwise normal. Symptomatic treatment for a few days is deemed adequate, while observing evolution of the disease that may be only a mild viral infection that may spontaneously resolve. Should the patient not improve, but his general condition remains stable, general blood and urine tests, a blood culture, and a chest X-ray are indicated; should these moderate-cost studies all be negative, empiric treatment with a broad-spectrum antibiotic can be started. Should the patient not respond, an intensive work-up to achieve an accurate final diagnosis would be indicated.

Example 2: A patient complains only of recent-onset cough. This could be a mild bronchitis treatable with a cough suppressant and expectorant. However, should the patient not recover soon, other diagnoses such as lung cancer must be considered.

Such cost-saving deferral of diagnosis risks missing the opportunity to cure a serious disease. For this reason, observation should be brief, carefully monitored, and the cost-benefit issue clearly understood by the patient.

Deferred diagnosis, empirical treatment, and other decisions required of a physician confronting disease are not readily translated into a computer algorithm. Providing the algorithm the necessary parameters—for example, patient age, general condition, potential seriousness of certain clinical data or diagnoses—might enable computer assistance with such decisions. The user is alerted to risk-flagged clinical data and diseases, and dangerous ("panic") laboratory values that could lead to a poor prognosis if not immediately addressed.

XVIII. DIAGNOSIS BY EXCLUSION

When clinical data of great PP value that strongly support a diagnosis are unavailable or too costly, the diagnostic process comes to a standstill. The physician then can resort to diagnosis by exclusion where, from a group of competing diagnoses, all but one are excluded. The single remaining diagnosis is accepted as a final diagnosis, even though its P is relatively small. With our double threshold method (page 87) for concluding the diagnostic quest, the P of such a diagnosis would not surpass the confirmation threshold and accordingly could not be legitimately considered as final, but instead would alone remain as non flagged in the differential diagnosis list. All other diagnoses would have been flagged as deleted because the great S of corresponding clinical data absent would have reduced their P below the deletion threshold. For example the diagnosis of acute appendicitis is acceptable when all other causes of acute right lower quadrant abdominal pain and tenderness have been excluded. The opposite of a diagnosis by exclusion would be a diagnosis supported by a pathognomonic or "clinching" clinical datum of great PP value that confers a high P to such an "assertive" diagnosis. An example is the diagnosis of tuberculosis when acid-fast bacilli are found in the sputum. Our algorithm automatically processes assertive and by exclusion diagnoses, once again illustrating the manner in which it emulates diagnosis by a physician.

XIX. COMPLEX CLINICAL PRESENTATIONS AND THEIR MODELS

Throughout the interaction between the physician and patient, involving medical examination, tests, and procedures, a jumble of clinical data is produced, which must be coalesced and organized into final diagnoses.

The diagnostic process comprises several levels of complexity. Related clinical data cluster to a syndrome, simple syndromes comprising only a few clinical data coalesce to a complex syndrome or disease, and sometimes to a yet more complex clinical presentation (page 12), where the relation of clinical data becomes less obvious.

The algorithm thus far presented uses **probabilistic** calculations, with mini-max procedure, best cost-benefit clinical datum, and discrimination between competing diagnoses and concurrent diagnoses, to determine the P of a final diagnosis. It will work well with simple clinical entities, such as uncomplicated diseases or syndromes where clinical data typically are interrelated and linked to a single cause or lesion. Examples of such simple diseases or clinical entities include bronchitis, asthma, gastroenteritis, hyperthyroidism, obstructive jaundice, and renal failure. At this diagnostic stage, a single final diagnosis accounts for all manifested clinical data. The accuracy of P depends on the accuracy of the S of clinical data. Determination of S (equation 2, page 24) with any method—retrospective, prospective, or estimative (page 24)—is labor intensive and requires the cooperation of a medical team. However, probabilistic calculations are feasible as long as they are applied to simple diseases or clinical entities, and statistically significant number of cases is available. The computational time of this stage is expected not to be excessive (non-exponential.)

In an actual patient, the clinical picture might be more complicated; as a fact, severely ill patients in intensive care units often have multi-organ involvement, present multiple and proteiform clinical data, and may mandate consultation with several specialists. For example, coronary artery disease, acute myocardial infarction, congestive heart failure, shock, *and* thromboembolism in a single patient. A specific disease can manifest diverse clinical forms and clinical presentations, complicating the diagnostic process. This situation makes impossible to determine the S of each clinical datum for the entire *complex clinical presentation* that involves multiple clinical forms, concurrent diseases, and multiple pathogenic and pathophysiologic mechanisms. It would require analyzing a statistically significant number of cases with identical combinations of clinical entities; it also would take us into an exponential or NP-complete computational time and complexity. Accordingly, probabilistic methods are unsuitable for processing *any* complex clinical presentation; indeed, to my knowledge, no commercial diagnostic programs that can accomplish this exist. A **categorical** method for processing complex clinical presentations is mandatory.

For this reason our algorithm, with its heuristic principles and moderate use of probability, diagnoses first only relatively simple syndromes, clinical entities, and diseases. Let the diagnostic algorithm produce as many final diagnoses of simple concurrent diseases, syndromes, complications, etc. as the clinical data dictate. Our algorithm is able to diagnose satisfactorily these simple clinical entities or diseases and also to recognize concurrency. Once we have these partial components (clinical entities), the knowledge base must offer categorical models (*clinical presentation models*; see below), one for each possible clinical interrelation or association of these entities: causal relations, stages, complications, severity, type, localization, etc. We believe that such clinical presentation models, although numerous, are not excessive, and are described in any authoritative medical textbook. The algorithm selects the clinical presentation model that accommodates best all the final clinical entities and diagnoses, probabilistically determined. It reminds me the jigsaw puzzles where different pieces must fit together in some meaningful way. This diagnostic stage does not require a probabilistic approach, but a pure categorical one.

Categorically relating clinical entities based on their associated pathophysiologic links or statistical correlations, into a complex clinical presentation mandate creating a specific model for each possible combination. We call these models complex clinical presentation models.

Complex clinical presentation model: a list of all diseases or clinical entities that are potentially related by pathophysiologic links or statistical correlations (examples in Fig. 11, next page.)

These examples are incomplete; not all linked clinical entities are shown. The direction of a causal link, when known, is indicated by an arrow. A complex clinical presentation model should comprise only clinical entities that present a close pathophysiologic relationship or clear statistical correlation. When a clinical entity (*e.g.*, atrial fibrillation in examples 1 and 2) appears in diverse complex clinical presentation models (*e.g.*, atrial fibrillation linked to myocardial infarction in one complex presentation model and linked to hyperthyroidism in another), such clinical entities should *not* be cross-linked. Dissimilar pathophysiologic mechanisms for such clinical entities may be involved in diverse presentation models. Such "trans-model" links (dotted lines in Fig. 11) would result in undesirable entangled networks (page 10-11), as encountered in some diagnostic programs, and which greatly complicate implementation, utilization, and updating. Of all clinical entities that appear in the complex presentation models, only final diagnoses (italicized in Example 1) determined in an actual patient are displayed at the conclusion of the diagnostic quest.

A *complex clinical presentation model* comprises related *clinical entities* and *diseases*; clinical data are excluded from this definition because they are elements of a *disease model*.

Integration of each complex clinical presentation model requires searching of the mentioned relationships in medical literature.

Should two or more final diagnoses be obtained, the question arises as to whether the respective diseases are related or unrelated. When a relationship cannot be established the diseases are *unrelated concurrent*. Example: tonsillitis and a uterine fibroid are unrelated concurrent diseases, because no known pathogenesis or pathophysiology relates them. When either a statistical correlation (mechanism

Examples of complex clinical presentation models:

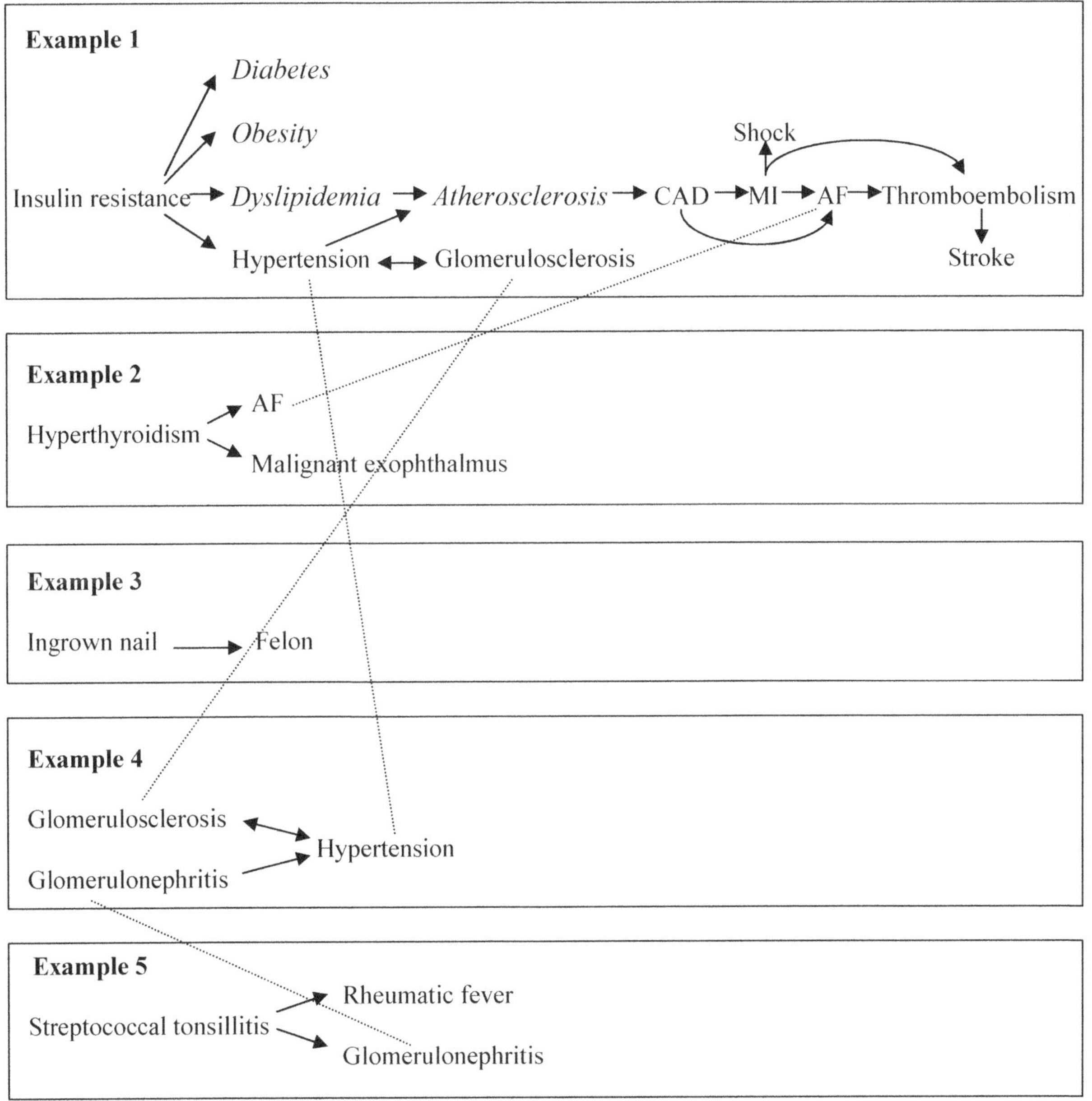

FIGURE 11. CAD, coronary artery disease; MI, myocardial infarction; AF, atrial fibrillation. Dotted lines represent *forbidden* cross-links between complex clinical presentation models (see text).

unknown) or pathophysiologic relationship can be established, we call these diseases *related concurrent* because actually they represent a single complex disease. An example is the metabolic syndrome that associates diabetes, obesity, dyslipidemia, hypertension, and vascular lesions. A statistical correlation among these diseases initially was observed; subsequent discovery of an underlying pathophysiologic common denominator (insulin receptor resistance) unified the apparently unrelated diseases to a complex clinical presentation. The knowledge base must be provided with *complex clinical presentation models* ideally listing all published *categorical* (as opposed to probabilistic) relations among clinical entities. When patient's final diagnoses of clinical entities fit into some of such complex clinical presentation models, they represent related concurrence; otherwise, they represent unrelated concurrence.

As mentioned earlier (page 11), many algorithms employ tree and network structures that extend from cause of disease to clinical data and *vice versa*, through several layers or levels, placing probabilities on nodes, branches, and leaves. Most such structures are complex and required years to assemble. I suspect that such structures are difficult to update and would need to be redesigned every few years. In contrast, our algorithm can relatively easily be updated at any time, by simply updating in disease models the S values of clinical data, adding or deleting clinical data when necessary, or adding or deleting disease models. Occasionally, the list of clinical entity combinations in the complex clinical presentation models must be modified when new associations are discovered. However, because the chain of clinical events linking cause of disease, lesions, clinical data, syndromes, and clinical presentation exists, we cannot completely ignore the tree or network structure. When required, as in clinical presentation models, we use these structures categorically, avoiding statistical and probabilistic calculations along their nodes, branches, and leaves. Complex clinical presentation models can be conceived as lists of causally or hierarchically related clinical entities, and not necessarily as trees or networks; in either form, we insist that they must be processed categorically, without any probabilistic component. A relational database can convert ("normalize") a tree or network to a list and *vice versa* [27]. Normalizing in database organization has a different meaning than the same term in probabilities (page 44.) Essential rule:

To be practical, the algorithm must not be too complex and the knowledge base must be relatively easy to implement and to update.

In summary, the entire diagnostic process is achieved in 2 steps:

Step 1. Probabilistic processing of clinical data

This step matches patient clinical data with disease model clinical data, yielding a differential diagnosis list. Mini-max procedure, best cost-benefit clinical data next to investigate, safety checks for interaction and risk identifiers, and discrimination between competing diagnoses and concurrent diagnoses achieve as many concurrent final diagnoses of clinical entities as are required to account for all manifested clinical data. Then, the algorithm proceeds to step 2.

Step 2. Categorical processing of clinical entities

Step 2.1. Safety checks to avoid overlooking related clinical entities: The algorithm applies a safety check that compares each final diagnosis (*e.g.*, pneumothorax) to all complex clinical presentation models in the knowledge base. Clinical entities related to pneumothorax (*e.g.*, tuberculosis, emphysema, or lung cancer) occurring in matching models are included in the differential diagnosis list to be processed for their presence or absence in the patient.

Step 2.2. Establishing related or unrelated concurrence of clinical entities: When two or more clinical entities are confirmed as final diagnoses, they are compared to all clinical presentation models in the knowledge base. When no complex clinical presentation model linking two or more clinical entities exists, such clinical entities are displayed as unrelated concurrent diagnoses, and the diagnostic quest concludes. When such a complex clinical presentation model exists the linked clinical entities are displayed as related concurrent, and the diagnostic quest concludes.

Several situations may occur when matching and selecting complex clinical presentation models:

- When more than one clinical presentation model is matched, that which links the greatest number of confirmed final diagnoses will be selected to account for the complex clinical presentation.

- When two or more clinical presentation models link a like number of confirmed final diagnoses, all such models will be selected as alternative representations of the complex clinical presentation.

- When diagnosed clinical entities match only some entities of the complex clinical presentation model, this nevertheless suffices to select the model and link the clinical entities. For example, not all complications listed in a single complex clinical presentation model need be matched; one complication (*e.g.*, pneumothorax) and one cause (*e.g.*, emphysema) suffice to link these two clinical entities.

- When one set of diagnosed clinical entities matches one clinical presentation model, while another set matches another clinical presentation model, the sets do not share clinical entities and the two clinical presentations are concurrent.

- When clinical presentation models involve clinical entities that are related in opposite directions (*e.g.*, myocardial infarction $\rightarrow$ shock; or shock $\rightarrow$ myocardial infraction), such alternatives are displayed and the user selects the direction that is most consistent with the clinical picture.

Essential rule:

An algorithm must be able to diagnose clinical forms and complex clinical presentations.

XX. HEURISTIC RESTRICTIVE TACTICS IN OUR ALGORITHM

Were we to exhaustively process all possible combinations of clinical data and all of approximately 4000 known diseases, 2^{4000} combinations would result; according to some estimate the resulting number is greater than the number of atoms that comprise the known universe. Therefore, to exhaustively process all diagnostic combinations is impossible; it would require a prohibitively long processing time (**computational time complexity**), mandating a heuristic reduction.

Excessive proliferation of clinical data and diagnoses to be processed, and inordinate iteration of complex mathematical equations may result in an exponential computation time creating an information flow bottleneck at the corresponding algorithm step. For these reasons, some computer programs limit the number of disease models by excluding very rare diseases and by basing diagnoses on a limited number of clinical data, thereby violating the essential rule that an algorithm must exhaustively consider all known diseases (page 27.)

Let's review some of the heuristic restrictive functions of our algorithm:

- Neither all described clinical data nor all known diseases contained in our knowledge base are exhaustively processed. Collection of all possible *none* and *small cost category* manifested clinical data and inclusion in the differential diagnosis list of all selected diagnoses are done only initially (see Initial Collection of Clinical Data on page 33.) This could produce an abundant, but not overwhelming amount of information.

- Should additional steps based on more costly tests or procedures be required to fine tune the differential diagnosis, the powerful heuristic restriction of the best cost-benefit clinical datum next to investigate function comes into play. This function searches only those clinical data with PP values and S values, which typically exceed those previously processed.

- Considering the greatest PP value of all clinical data supporting a diagnosis, as the P of the diagnosis (equation 6, page 40) seems to function well, avoiding inaccuracies and complicated calculations.

- The mini-max procedure (page 39) has important heuristic properties that enable calculation of diagnostic probabilities and identification and processing of concurrent diseases.

- Our categorical method for dealing with complex clinical presentations and causal relationships of clinical entities (page 91) circumvents the prolonged and cumbersome probability calculations involved in other methods.

- Safety checks, empirical treatment, deferred diagnosis, and diagnosis by exclusion also may be considered heuristic restrictive tactics.

- Our algorithm calculates the PP value of each clinical datum for each known disease, involving considerable computer time. However, these operations are done only once by the manufacturer, before the program is delivered, as opposed to real time calculation during the diagnostic process. With our algorithm, operations done in real time during a diagnostic quest involve matching patient clinical data with those in all disease models. Although a great number of disease models exist, computational time is polynomial, as opposed to exponential; modern computational methods abbreviate this process. A similar situation occurs during the selection process of the best cost-benefit clinical datum, where a great number of clinical data not yet considered must be selected from the disease models, but are restricted to diagnoses already in the differential diagnosis list. Only clinical data with great PP value and S are processed. The type and number of operations involved in calculating probabilities of diagnoses in the differential diagnosis list with the 3-Step method of the best cost-benefit clinical datum procedure are described on pages 58, 59, and 61.

COMMENTS

ACCURACY OF OUR ALGORITHM

In the following paragraphs we will discuss on what factors the accuracy of our algorithm relies.

Our algorithm, like many others, is based on clinical data *sensitivity* (S). Accordingly, the accuracy of our final diagnosis substantially depends on the statistical accuracy of these S, which in turn depends on the number of clinical cases analyzed. To determine the sensitivity of each clinical datum, Perlroth and Weiland [17], reviewed 1000 cases of each of 50 diseases. The more cases that are analyzed, the more accurate will be S. The sensitivity also relies on the carefulness with which the reporting physician studies each patient, so as not to overlook a clinical datum present. The sensitivity of a clinical datum also may depend on the patient's age, race, sex, and on environmental factors. The algorithm must be tested to ascertain whether minor accuracy variability of S is critical or may be disregarded.

Completeness of disease models and complex clinical presentation models.

The *number of clinical data collected* may also influence the diagnostic accuracy. This again emphasizes the importance of an adequate history and physical examination. The more clinical data collected, the less the likelihood of missing a disease. Investigation of additional clinical data adds to the cost and time involved. When the search for clinical data in the low cost category has been exhausted, we typically must progress to costlier categories, where data with greater PP value or S values often are found. This again reminds me of a kind of receiver operating characteristic (ROC) curve: the more clinical data searched, the more accurate the diagnosis, but the greater the cost. On the other hand, we need not search the entire PP value and S lists, but only focus on clinical data of great PP value or S value. The algorithm could display only the most significant clinical data of the PP value list and S list and hide those that are less discriminative. How many clinical data need to be displayed can be determined by practical experience.

Another important ROC curve type of tuning the diagnostic process depends on the *magnitude assigned to the thresholds* that determine the conclusion of the diagnostic quest (page 87.) Because our algorithm virtually emulates actual diagnostic situations, it can be tuned by empirically decreasing or increasing the mentioned parameters, then observe how its accuracy compares to that of the human diagnosis.

We want to close the above considerations with a philosophical meditation. Many mental processes or decision-making actions seem to follow the ROC curve. The more advantages we want to gain in life, the more we must pay in terms such as price, suffering, risk, and expended time. Perfection is unlikely to be achieved in diagnosis, prognosis, or therapeusis, whether or not a computer is involved. For this reason, many criticisms and malpractice suits against physicians often are unfair.

UNCERTAINTIES OF OUR ALGORITHM

A computer program based on our algorithm that can be challenged with actual patient examples has not yet been written. For this reason, we decided to test the algorithm manually. In general, this effort was successful, but revealed some weaknesses that were corrected. Uncertainties that remain include:

- How critical is to take into consideration the *qualities of certain clinical data*? (Page 22.)

- *Comprehensive initial data collection versus gradual built up* (comprehensive and abridged methods, page 34.)

- How much *proliferation of information* will the successive collections of clinical data and diagnoses create? (Page 37 and 57.)

- What is the validity of considering the *highest PP value* of clinical data supporting a diagnosis equal to the P of that diagnosis? (Page 40.)

- Is considering the *greatest S* of absent clinical data equivalent to maximal diagnostic rule-out power? (Pages 41) In some cases, absent clinical data of smaller S can still decrease the P of a diagnosis; in other cases, absent clinical data may increase the P. See property 4 of the mini-max procedure on page 51 and 3-Step procedure on page 58.

- Will the *diagnosis that accounts for the most clinical data* be the same as the *diagnosis of greatest probability*? (Page 38.)

- Magnitude of *cut off point in ROC curve for thresholds ending the diagnostic quest* (page 87.)

- Which is the *best method of concluding the diagnostic quest*? (Page 87.)

- How efficient will be the *set of best cost-benefit clinical data* simultaneously recommended? (Page 63.)

- Is the preferred mini-max method or an alternative method the best for identifying and selecting *concurrent diseases*? (Page 85-86.)

- How will the matching of clinical entities with *complex clinical presentation models* function? (Page 91.)

- Should concurrent diagnoses be processed in a *single* or *separate differential diagnoses lists*; if required, when should separation occur? (Page 85.)

- *How critical is sensitivity accuracy*, considering its variance with clinical presentation, age, sex, race, environment, author, etc.? (Page 97.)

- How reliable are *safety checks* such as risk and interaction identifiers to preclude missing important diagnoses? (Page 89.)

A prototype program should provide answers to these questions. A limited number of disease models can then be created and the program challenged with actual simple and complex clinical cases.

NOVEL CONCEPTS OF OUR ALGORITHM

Our diagnostic program includes novel ideas not mentioned in the extensive literature references reviewed. Some of the ideas are original in themselves; others are original based on a special manner in which extant elements are combined.

- *Disregarding disease prevalence* (page 23) is doubly advantageous: (1) Prior probabilities of diseases (equivalent to prevalence) are eliminated from Bayes formula, which is transformed into a simplified equation 5 for calculating the PP value from statistically established S values of clinical data (page 26.) (2) Low prevalence no longer is a cause of excluding a rare disease from a differential diagnosis list, giving this disease a chance to become a final diagnosis, based on merit of supporting clinical data.

- *Disregarding subjective qualities of clinical data* (page 22), which are variable and unreliable, remarkably simplifies diagnostic processing without losing accuracy.

- We believe that the *PP value best indicates how strongly a clinical datum supports a diagnosis and more accurately* than does specificity, true positive value, estimated evoking strength [13] [24], or any other index attached to a clinical datum; its value does not change unless the sensitivities of clinical data are changed (page 25.)

- *PP values can be calculated and included in the knowledge base before the diagnostic program is delivered to the user*, avoiding real time calculation.

- Considering the *greatest of the PP values of clinical data present that support a diagnosis, equal to the P of this diagnosis* would appear superior to arithmetically combining values of several redundant supportive clinical data, thereby inappropriately increasing the P of the diagnosis (page 39.)

- Our *mini-max procedure* (page 39) for determining the P of a diagnosis overcomes the deficiencies of the typical Bayes formula. In a novel way, the algorithm combines a modified weight averaging Bayes formula (page 44) with the mini-max principle, to calculate the P of a diagnosis. Original Bayes formula processes sequentially or simultaneously *multiple* clinical data present and absent. Because these clinical data are interrelated, this application violates the independence and incompatibility principles (page 27), leading to inaccuracies of calculated P. We apply Bayes averaged formula only to a *single* clinical datum present and a *single* clinical datum absent, in each clinical data pair, which does not violate those principles, and we eliminate prior probability of diseases from it. Once the partial P conferred to the diagnoses by each of all possible clinical data pairs are calculated with the modified averaging Bayes formula, they are integrated into a total P by the mini-max procedure. In this manner, we obtain the benefit of two worlds: original Bayes formula is inaccurate for multiple clinical data processing, but accurate for single pairs of one clinical datum present and one clinical datum absent. Mini-max principle alone does not take into account the appropriate proportional significance of S that is considered by the weight averaged Bayes formula; however, it is appropriate to integrate the partial P values calculated by this formula into a total P of the diagnosis.

- At each step of the diagnostic inquiry, we apply a novel method to select and recommend the *best cost-benefit clinical datum next to investigate* (page 53), which heuristically reduces the number of new clinical data searched, thereby considerably shortening the diagnostic process. Unlike other diagnostic programs, our algorithm considers greatest PP value, S, and cost in selecting the best cost-benefit clinical datum.

- *Cost has high priority* in our program (page 62) and refers not only to the dollar *price*, but also to *discomfort* and *risk*; the maximum of these qualitative levels represents the overall cost (page 29.)

- *Simultaneously recommending several best cost-benefit clinical data* (page 63) provides a novel and important advantage over recommending only one at each diagnostic step.

- Ability of our mini-max procedure to *distinguish competitive diagnoses from concurrent diagnoses* (page 81.)

- Conclusion of diagnostic quest is treated in a manner similar to that used by other authors. However, I have not found literature references to the creation of *confirmation* and *deletion thresholds* as we describe on page 87.

- The *entire diagnostic process is partitioned into two distinct steps* (page 94): the first step uses *probabilities* to obtain final diagnoses; the second step uses *categorical* tools to preclude overlooking related clinical entities and to establish unrelated or related concurrency among diagnosed clinical entities, integrating them into complex clinical presentations. This partitioning eliminates the computational complexity and even impossibility of managing the entire diagnostic process with probabilistic calculations.

- *Risk identifiers, interaction identifiers, and other safety checks* (page 89)—to preclude overlooking important diagnoses—as well as *empirical treatment, diagnosis by exclusion, and deferred diagnosis* are also important heuristic aspects that complete the benefits of our algorithm.

- The knowledge base must be integrated with all known disease models, including sensitivity (PP values are automatically calculated) and cost category of each clinical datum, risk and interaction identifiers, empirical values for confirmation and deletion thresholds, and all known complex clinical presentation models. When clinical data present and absent are provided, the algorithm is expected to return accurate final diagnoses and complex clinical presentations in an almost automatic manner.

Our diagnostic program could be expanded to include prognostic and therapeutic guidelines. A more ambitious project might be to determine whether other inexact disciplines such as law, sociology, politics, defense, or corporate strategy could benefit from some steps of our algorithm.

SOME "PHILOSOPHICAL" MEDITATIONS

During the diagnostic process, one can observe the fascinating interplay between machine, human and social factors, and the physical reality of the patient.

The computer working at a speed of gigahertz, processing a great number of clinical data, clinical entities, and diagnoses, tends to produce a huge proliferation of information, which is swiftly contained by restrictive heuristic tactics.

Then, the resulting information is presented to the physician who should discuss it with the patient, at a humanitarian pace. Here socio-economic circumstances will play a role in the physician and patient acceptance of the proposed next step when it involves a more costly test or procedure. The maximum cost limit depends on patient age and sex, willingness to undergo the procedure, financial status, insurance coverage and approval, environmental risks, and many other factors.

The physical reality of the patient's body will decide the result, positive or negative, of the test or procedure.

The result is entered in the computer and the machine-physician-patient-society cycle is iterated. Each new clinical datum, with its presence or absence in the patient, sets a new stage for the next datum selection until final diagnoses are achieved, cost exceeds benefit, or all clinical data are exhausted.

Clinical practice involves many subtleties that a physician learns from experience rather than from theory. A diagnostic program based on human reasoning and skills should emulate these nuances. This requires a thorough review of clinical practice in its entirety, discovering such nuances that we hope are not excessive in number. Researchers lack of time and patience, needed to carry out such review, could be a major reason why a patient's bedside successful diagnostic computer program has not been achieved until now. Several of these nuances were addressed, discussed, and processed in this research; probably some others remain unnoticed. A sustained effort to unveil such nuances will enable us to perfect the algorithm.

So far, we have analyzed the amazing assistance that computers provide, based on their vast storage capacities and great processing speeds. However, let's not forget that many other tasks cannot be handled by computers. To obtain reliable and comprehensive clinical data, a careful history taking (a checklist filled out by the patient is an imperfect alternative) and a thorough physical examination must be done by a physician. Recall the classical saying regarding computers: "garbage in, garbage out". Having been trained at my medical school in the collection of clinical data through a subject called *Semiology* (semeion = symptoms; logos = study) that was taught every morning during the entire academic year, I find very contrasting how neglected this subject is in some other medical schools. I must admit that things have changed dramatically over the past 50 years in light of the astonishing new diagnostic technologies that greatly replaced some of the old practices. Even so, some traditional symptoms and signs remain essential, at least for the initial diagnostic orientation, and should not be taught by voluntary general practitioners as seen in some university hospitals.

Furthermore, the best cost-benefit clinical datum next to investigate recommended by the algorithm, including its significance and possible outcome must be explained to and discussed with the patient, especially if a costlier procedure is involved. Patient-physician rapport, recommendations, clarifications, and often human understanding, humility, sympathy, reassurance, compassion, hope, consolation, and solutions to ethical problems obviously cannot be provided by a computer.

A final thought for this section: When I initially conceived a diagnostic computer program half a century ago, physicians were overwhelmed with learning and remembering a virtually endless number of diseases, syndromes, symptoms, signs, and diverse maneuvers for inspecting, palpating, percussing, and auscultating organs, etc. Scientific and technical advances such as computed tomography, sonography, MRI, radioimmunoassay, flexible endoscopy, DNA testing, cloning, among others, shifted the attention of clinicians from patient contact to modern laboratory technology.

When will we reach a Utopian future where a patient is analyzed by a machine that scans all his organs, determines whether they are functioning normally or abnormally, determines his genetic endowment, delivers an accurate diagnosis without asking a single question, then sends a bill? I ask myself whether a diagnostic program such as ours is still needed.

My answer to this question is that, in the first place, the mentioned Utopia seems distant, if ever possible. In the second place, even though techniques, procedures, and knowledge will evolve, thousands of diseases will continue to exist; the enormous amount of associated information will be manageable only with computers. Algorithms based on the general principles described in this essay almost certainly will remain useful.

CONCLUSIONS

Our algorithm, although somewhat complex, is straightforward, especially when compared to other attempts in this field. It emulates a clinician's diagnostic reasoning. It is logical and mathematically simple. Bayes formula is used with modifications, because it is unable to process properly interdependent clinical data (as are most symptoms) and concurrent diseases. To facilitate implementation and updating of the algorithm, we tend to avoid complicated tools of artificial intelligence, such as causal, hierarchical, and probabilistic trees and networks. The algorithm freely uses heuristic procedures, so as to preclude excessive proliferation of clinical data and diagnoses. It promises to be user friendly because it is expressed in natural language, is rational, and readily understandable. It also is readily translatable to a computer program; we provide a flowchart of the algorithm that includes all steps of the diagnostic process. Determination of accurate sensitivity of clinical data and integration of clinical entities into clinical presentation models will be labor-intensive. As soon as a prototype program proves the concept viable, a complete knowledge base with all known diseases, clinical data, clinical presentations, and other information can be created. This major task will require a dedicated team. Establishing the sensitivity of all clinical data for all known diseases will be especially time-consuming. This could be accomplished by (a) retrospectively incorporating information from past medical records and publications; (b) prospectively incorporating information from future medical records. The latter task would be an ongoing project, but would be facilitated by universal electronic storage and processing of medical records; (c) basing the sensitivities on the personal estimation of clinicians and specialists, but this is subjective and inaccurate. The expected great benefits of such a medical resource are worth the effort. Perhaps it could be compared with the team effort invested by the creators of many existing multi-volume dictionaries or encyclopedias, or the implementation of some extensive information systems over the Internet.

For many years, I have conceived as an **important project** the creation of a database, whether or not used in a computer program, with two parts. In the first part, all known *diseases* will be listed alphabetically, each with all its corresponding clinical data indexed with S and PP value, in the manner of Perlroth and Weiland [17] (page 21.) This part equates to our *disease models*; it would provide at a glance all clinical data that a disease can manifest and how strongly each clinical datum supports (PP value of clinical datum present) or denies (S of clinical datum absent) a diagnosis. The second part, reciprocally arranged, will alphabetically list all known *clinical data* (with synonyms), each with all the diseases (again with corresponding S and PP values), that can manifest this clinical datum. This part equates to our *clinical datum lists*, enabling the health care provider to see at a glance which diseases can account for a specific clinical datum, and with what frequency (S value) and strength (PP value.)

We mentioned (page 21), that physicians typically are unsatisfied with knowing only final diagnoses. They want to know the causes of diseases and the syndromes that bridge causes or lesions with clinical data. Information concerning disease etiology, pathogenesis, pathology, pathophysiology, syndromes, complications, clinical presentation models, prognosis, and treatment can be retrieved from the knowledge base. To facilitate study and research, general medical information with selected references to the literature should be provided.

The evolution of computerized medical diagnosis has explored four main idea paths: 1. Pattern recognition. 2. Bayesian probabilities. 3. Networks based on pathogenic, pathophysiologic, and hierarchical relationships among diseases, lesions, and clinical data. 4. Diverse mathematical expressions that, to me and possibly to other clinicians, appear esoteric, totally inadequate for emulating human medical reasoning, and incapable of representing the many peculiar nuances involved in the diagnostic process. In an effort to unify these diverse paths, our algorithm integrates the best of these worlds. Our algorithm begins with pattern recognition, where patient clinical data are compared with disease model clinical data. Matching disease models are selected as diagnoses to be processed in a differential diagnosis list. Some researchers call these selected diagnoses *hypotheses*; we prefer to call them, in a more traditional clinical language, potential diagnoses, differential diagnoses, or simply diagnoses. The number of selected diagnoses might be great, but not overwhelming, and the processing time would be comparable to the time required by a computer to look up a limited number of words in an electronic dictionary.

The next task of the algorithm is to determine the relative probability of each competing diagnosis. In our opinion, accurate and efficient determination of such probabilities must utilize statistical and probabilistic tools in a limited manner, while avoiding typical, almost dogmatic use of Bayes formula. A salient problem—the lack of independence of the clinical data manifested by a disease—is a shortcoming of the Bayes formula when applied to calculation of the probability of a diagnosis [13]. To obviate this problem, some authors add, average, or multiply supporting clinical data values to obtain a final score that represents the relative probability of the diagnosis. Myers, Pople, and Miller [13] remark that some clinical data of a syndrome are somewhat redundant, in which case any of the aforementioned scoring methods would erroneously increase the probability of a diagnosis. To overcome this problem, we consider the highest PP value of all the clinical data present that support a diagnosis equal to the probability of the diagnosis, which to us seems reasonable and precludes laborious calculations.

Pople, Myers, and Miller [28] noted the importance of clinical data absent in reducing the probability of a diagnosis, which is inversely related to the sensitivity of these data. Our novel mini-max procedure simultaneously considers the effects of clinical data present and absent on the probability of a diagnosis.

Networks and logical trees offer interesting tools to represent pathogenic and pathophysiologic relations in the genesis of a disease. However, when the number of their levels increases and furthermore if their nodes, branches, and leaves bear probabilities (Bayesian networks) the attempt to implement the entire diagnostic process in form of networks becomes very messy and unpractical. Compounding this problem, ultimate pathogenic and phathophysiologic relationships are often unknown and the corresponding probabilities difficult to establish. Even were such networks created, they would require exhaustive search through an exponential number of probabilistic combinations.

At best, networks are useful when applied to closely-related clinical entities, in a purely categorical Boolean manner without probabilistic calculations. Bayesian networks collapse with complex, concurrent combinations of clinical entities or associations of diseases. Perhaps, similar remarks also would apply to algorithms based on production rules [29] and algorithms based exclusively on pattern recognition and probabilities.

In recent years, medical applications of computer research have been focused on algorithms dealing with time-related clinical data [4]. To establish a possible relationship (causal or stages of disease) between two clinical events, it is necessary to know the order of occurrence and the elapsed time interval. Because our algorithm operates in a cross-sectional manner, freezing time at a specific diagnostic moment, we have the impression that time is not critical, although significant time or sequence relations of clinical data or diagnoses can be integrated in the disease models and clinical presentation models, where appropriate.

SUMMARY OF ESSENTIAL RULES FOR A DIAGNOSTIC PROGRAM

To be efficient, accurate, and practical, a diagnostic computer program must fulfill some essential rules or requirements. Cross-references to the pages that explain these rules in detail are provided.

A diagnostic algorithm must essentially be based on categorical reasoning, with the fewest possible mathematical calculations, and provide cross-references to additional information such as etiology, pathogenesis, pathology, pathophysiology, syndromes, etc. (page 21.)

Disregard clinical data qualities in computer diagnosis programs (page 23.)

Disregard prevalence or prior probability of diseases in computer diagnosis programs (page 23.)

For clinical data, use standard terms or synonyms that are recognized by the algorithm (page 23.)

Do not assign sensitivity (S) to a syndrome, but only to its corresponding clinical data and let the algorithm calculate the probability (P) of such syndrome (page 25.)

To be accurate, a computer program must include and process *all* known diseases (page 27.)

Do *not* use Bayes formula to calculate the probability of a diagnosis (page 27.)

A clinical datum present rules in the corresponding diagnosis with strength proportional to its positive predictive value (PP value). A clinical datum absent rules out the corresponding diagnosis with strength proportional to its sensitivity (S) (page 32.)

A diagnostic algorithm must neither miss correct diagnoses nor recommend inappropriate or unnecessarily costly clinical data (page 35.)

An efficient algorithm must distinguish competing diagnoses from concurrent diseases (page 35.)

The probability (P) of a diagnosis equals the greatest positive predictive value (PP value) of the clinical data that support this diagnosis (page 40.)

An important function of a diagnostic algorithm is to inform at each diagnostic step, the most useful clinical datum next to investigate, considering cost versus benefit (page 53.)

To be practical for diagnosing actual cases, it is essential that a computerized diagnostic program be able to simultaneously recommend a *set* of best cost-benefit clinical data next to investigate (page 63.)

An efficient computer program must detect interactions among diseases and drugs (page 88.)

To be practical, the algorithm must not be too complex and the knowledge base must be relatively easy to implement and to update (page 94.)

An algorithm must be able to diagnose clinical forms and complex clinical presentations (page 95.)

APPENDIX A: KNOWLEDGE BASE AND ALGORITHM

I. KNOWLEDGE BASE

A preliminary task is to assemble the knowledge base.

Create a disease model (page 12) for each currently known clinical entity and disease, including models for health, death, and iatrogenic diseases. Each model comprises all clinical data that the disease can potentially manifest, with their corresponding indices—S, PP value, and cost—and identifiers—risk and interaction. When such indices and identifiers vary with age, gender, race, occupation, or any other demographic factor, the disease model should include such variations or a different disease model for each condition should be created.

Disease models and *clinical datum lists* are conveniently visualized and managed by entering in an huge virtual table (Table 3), the several thousand known diseases in the heading row, and the several thousand known clinical data in the first column.

Cost +...++++	Tuberculosis *	Bronchitis
Cough +	S = 0.83 PP value = 0.7	S = 0.95 PP value = 0.8
Hemoptisis + *	S = 0.7 PP value = 0.55	S = 0.05 PP value = 0.01
Dyspnea + *	S = 0.5 PP value = 0.4	
Fever + &		

TABLE 3. S, sensitivity; PP value, positive predictive value; +, no cost; ++, small cost; +++, intermediate cost; ++++, great cost; * risk identifier; &, interaction identifier

The cell, in which each diagnosis and its corresponding clinical datum converge, shows the S and PP value of the clinical datum for the disease. Many cells will show S = 0 and PP value = 0, meaning that the clinical datum never is manifested by the disease; these "empty" cells can be disregarded. After disregarding empty cells, each column represents a *disease model* and each row represents a potential *clinical datum list*. Each clinical datum shows its *cost* category with plus (+) signs. *Risk identifiers* are flagged with an asterisk (*). *Interaction identifiers* are flagged with an ampersand (&) in the cells of clinical data potentially modifiable by drugs or concurrent diseases.

During the matching process of patient clinical data present with clinical data in the disease models, the algorithm scans each clinical datum row, sorting out matched diseases that show an S or PP value > 0, creating a corresponding *clinical datum list*. Clinical data present in the patient are stored. Later in the diagnostic process, the algorithm will scan the column of each disease model corresponding to diagnoses included in differential diagnosis list, sorting out clinical data not yet investigated. These clinical data comprise the *PP value and S lists*, from which the *best cost-benefit clinical datum next to investigate* will be selected (page 53).

Create *complex clinical presentations models* for all possible combinations of clinical entities and diseases (page 91.)

Create a routine that enables updating of the knowledge base. When a new disease is discovered, the corresponding disease model must be added to the knowledge base. When, for a known disease, a new clinical datum is established with a novel test or procedure, it must be included in the corresponding disease model. As clinical data referring to new cases of known diseases become available, S and PP values must be updated.

Create a dictionary with common synonyms for clinical data (page 23.)

Calculate the PP value of every clinical datum, based on the S values, according to equation 5 (page 26.)

Create four clinical data cost categories: none, small, intermediate, and great (page 29.) Estimate the cost of obtaining each clinical datum and assign this datum to the corresponding category.

Flag risky clinical data and diagnoses (see risk identifiers, pages 30 and 89.)

Flag clinical data, the S of which can be modified by concurrent diseases or drug interactions. List such diseases and drugs for corresponding clinical data (see interaction identifiers, page 88.)

In the knowledge base, for each diagnosis create cross-references to the corresponding cause of the disease, pathogenesis, pathology, pathophysiology, syndromes, complications, stages, interactions with other diseases and drugs, prognosis and treatment, and any other pertinent information related to the disease.

Establish empiric values for confirmation and deletion thresholds (page 87.) Such values must be empirically determined by comparing actual clinical cases with computer performance; however, they must be adjustable to the circumstances of the specific case—diagnostic uncertainty, disease severity, evolution, prognosis, and efficacious treatment availability.

Provide routines to update or edit any information in the knowledge base.

II. ALGORITHM AND FLOWCHARTS

In this section, we summarize the principal steps that comprise our diagnostic algorithm.

FIGURE 1. Summary flowchart of diagnostic algorithm

The diagnostic algorithm executes successive steps via several routines (Figs. 2 through 19.)

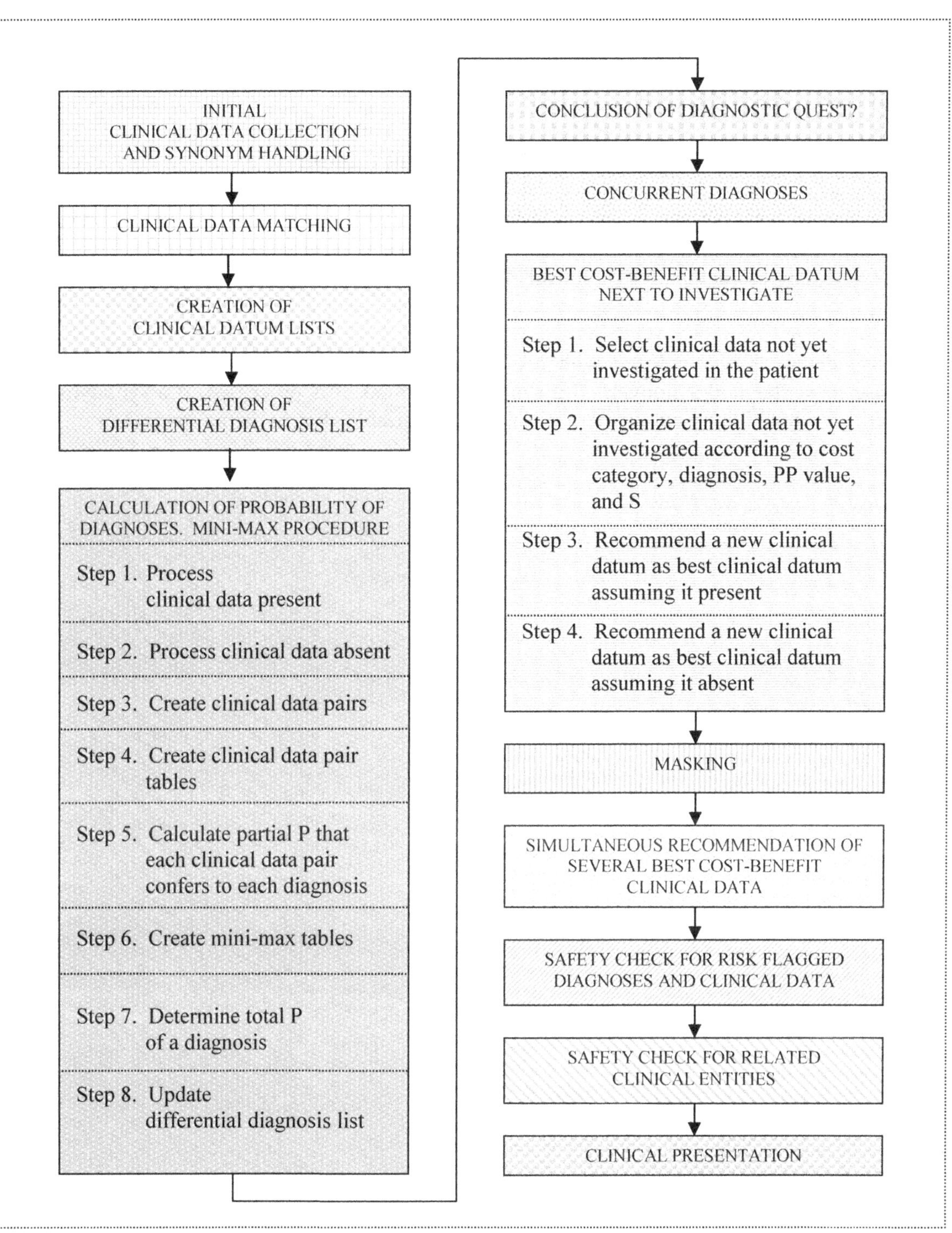

FIGURE 1. SUMMARY FLOWCHART OF DIAGNOSTIC ALGORITHM

ROUTINE FLOWCHARTS OF DIAGNOSTIC ALGORITHM
(Based on preferred methods described in the text)

FIGURE 2. Initial clinical data collection and synonym handling

Provide the computer with patient general information, followed by initially collected clinical data (page 33.) Prompt user to indicate whether each clinical datum is present or absent. Clinical data present will create clinical datum lists; clinical data absent are stored for future use in ruling out diagnoses.

When a clinical datum is not matched with a clinical datum in any disease model, search in the knowledge base for a standard synonym. If a synonym is found, it is processed; if a synonym is not found, the user is prompted to try another term for the unidentifiable clinical datum (page 23.)

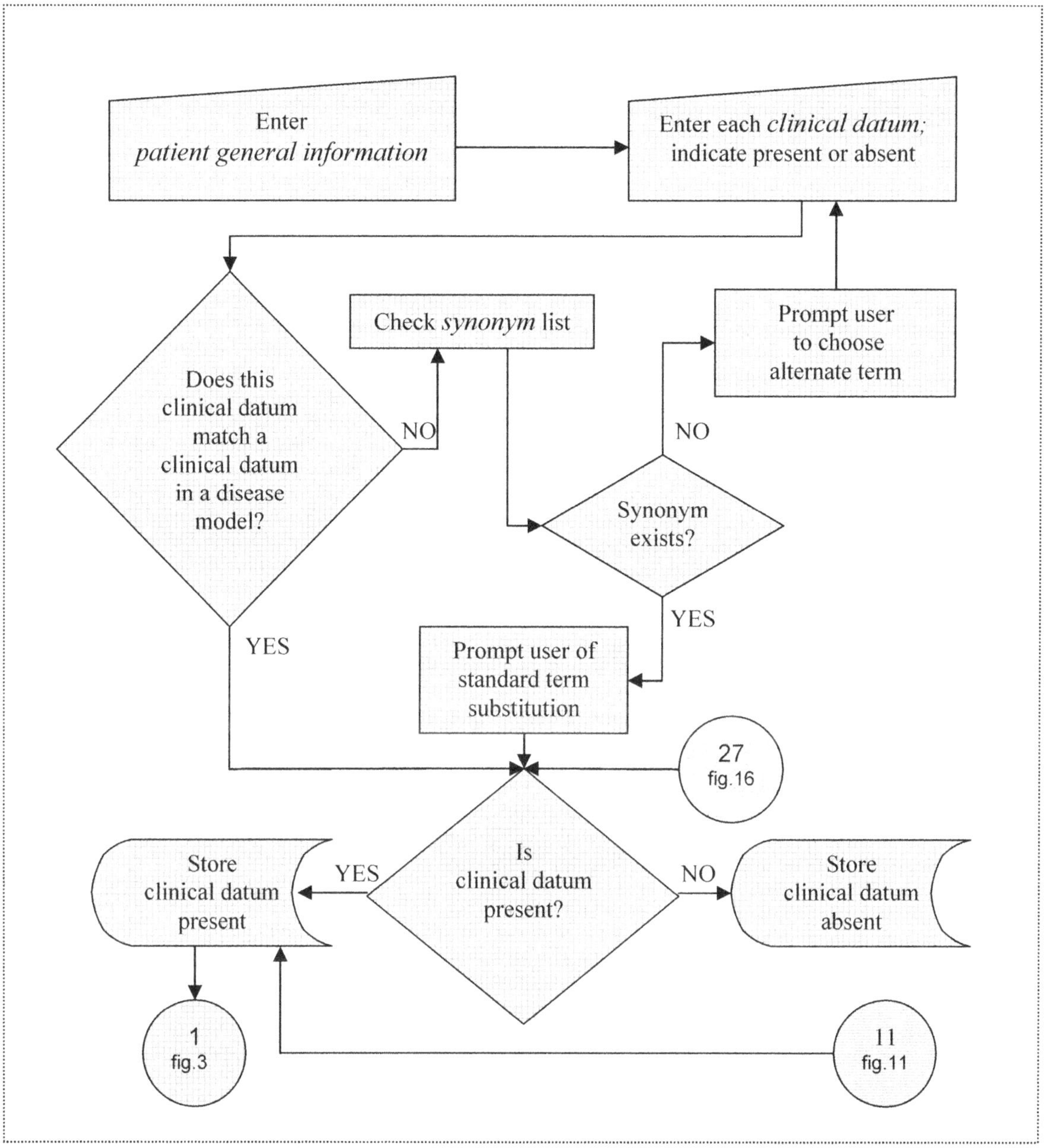

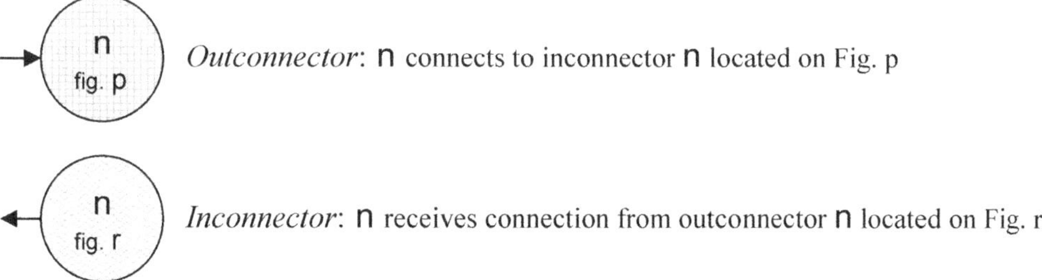

FIGURE 2. INITIAL CLINICAL DATA COLLECTION AND SYNONYM HANDLING

FIGURE 3. Matching of collected clinical data present with clinical data in disease models

Compare each clinical datum present with clinical data listed in each disease model; select all disease models (diagnoses) that show a match (page 35.)

FIGURE 4. Creation of clinical datum lists

Create a clinical datum list headed by the name of the clinical datum present and listing all diagnoses that could manifest such datum; arrange S and PP values of this clinical datum for each diagnosis by decreasing numerical value (page 35.)

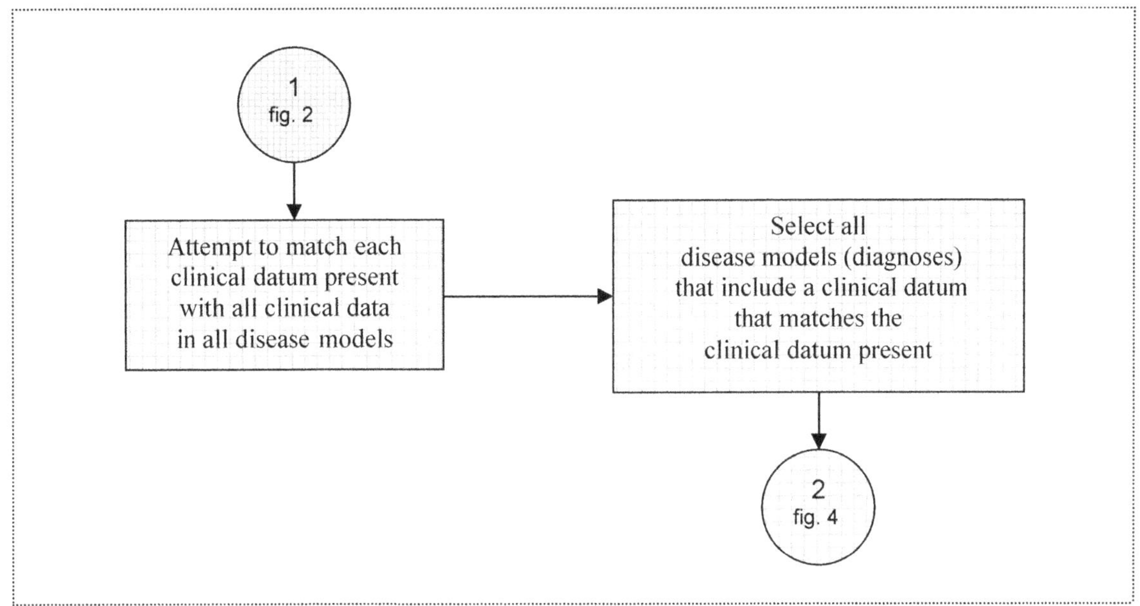

FIGURE 3. CLINICAL DATA MATCHING

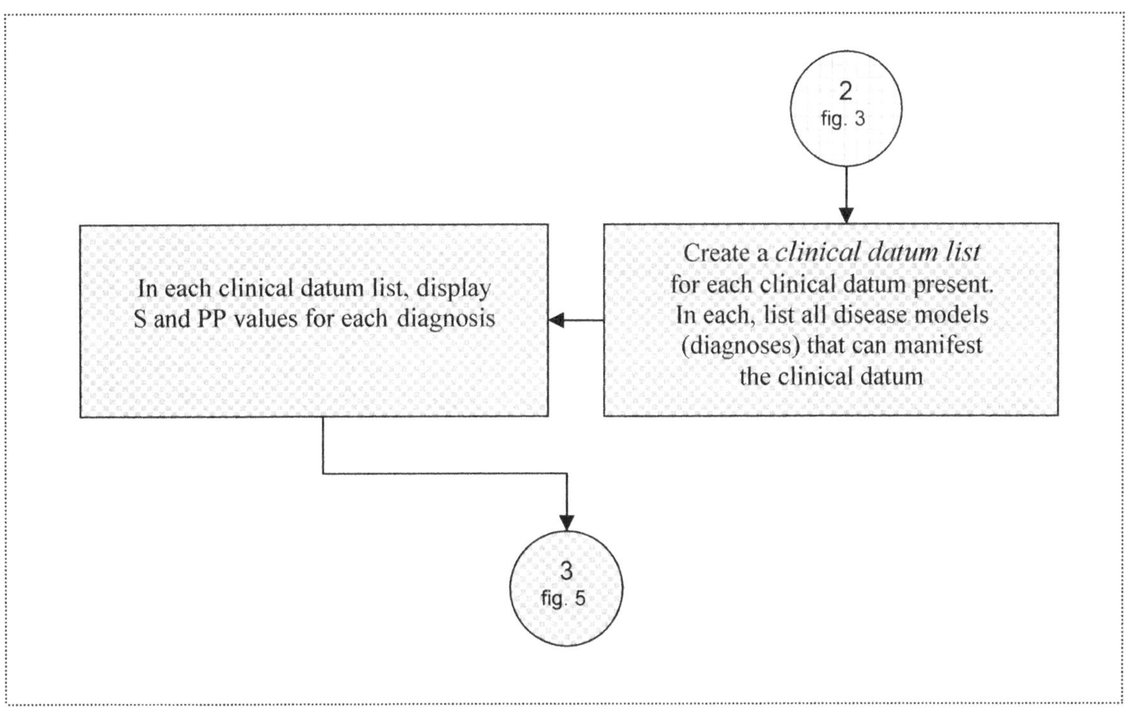

FIGURE 4. CREATION OF CLINICAL DATUM LISTS

FIGURE 5. Creation of differential diagnosis list

Create a differential diagnosis list that includes all diagnoses appearing in all clinical datum lists without repeating diagnoses (all-inclusive method, page 37.)

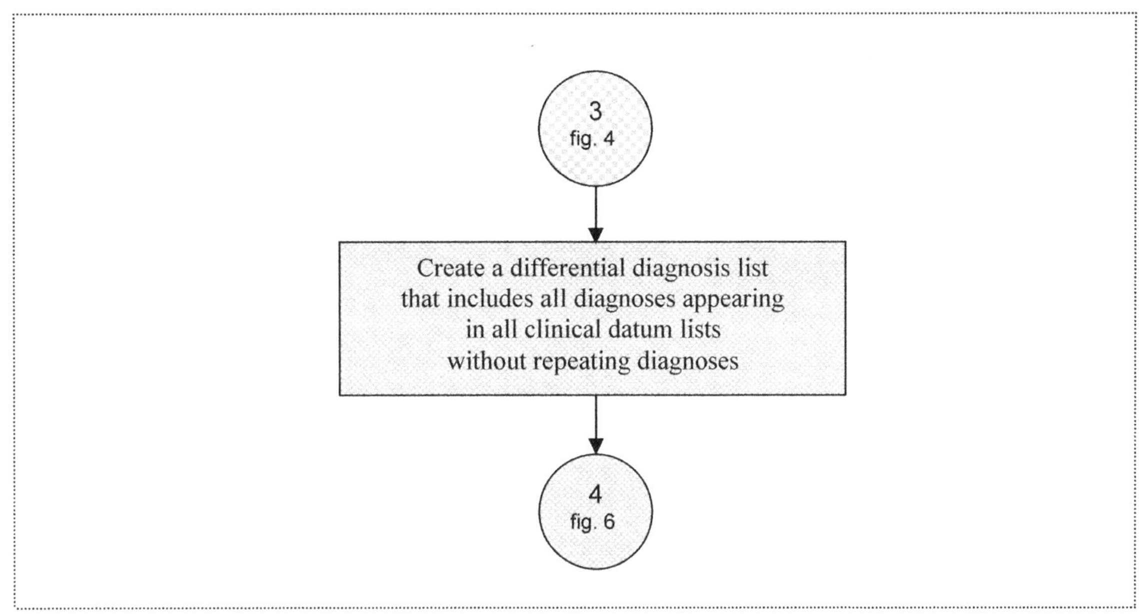

FIGURE 5. CREATION OF DIFFERENTIAL DIAGNOSIS LIST

FIGURES 6 through 9. Probability of diagnoses. Mini-max procedure

FIGURE 6

Step 1. *Process clinical data present.* For each diagnosis in the differential diagnosis list, select from the set of clinical datum lists the clinical datum with the greatest PP value that supports *this* diagnosis (page 40.) The selected greatest PP value equals the P of this diagnosis. This value can be modified by clinical data absent (next step).

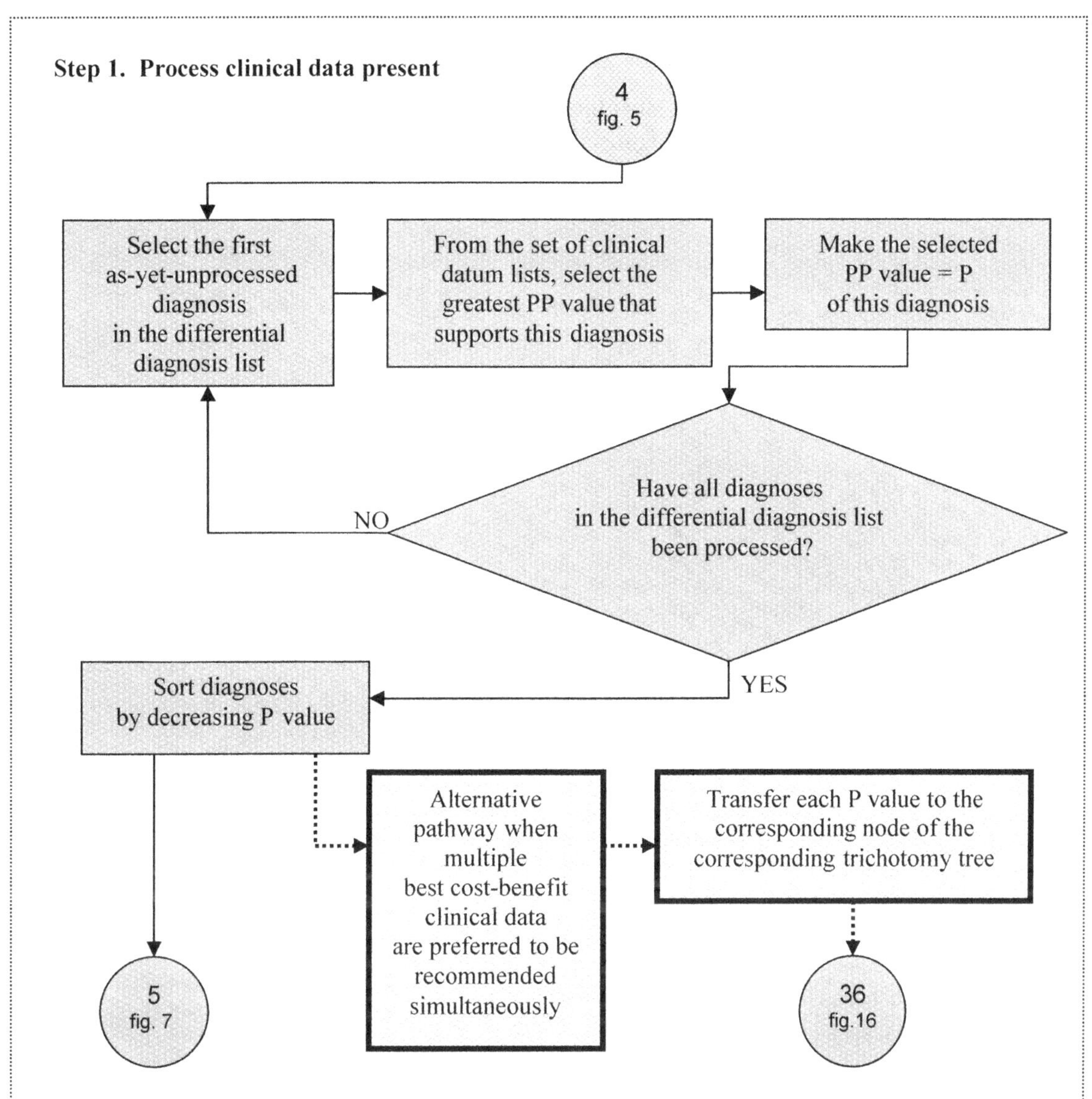

FIGURE 6. CALCULATION OF PROBABILITY OF DIAGNOSES. MINI-MAX PROCEDURE

Step 2. *Process clinical data absent.* Delete clinical data absent (obtained from patient history) that do not refer to diagnoses in the differential diagnosis list (page 41.)

Step 3. *Create clinical data pairs.* Create clinical data pairs comprising all possible combinations of one clinical datum present and one clinical datum absent (page 44.)

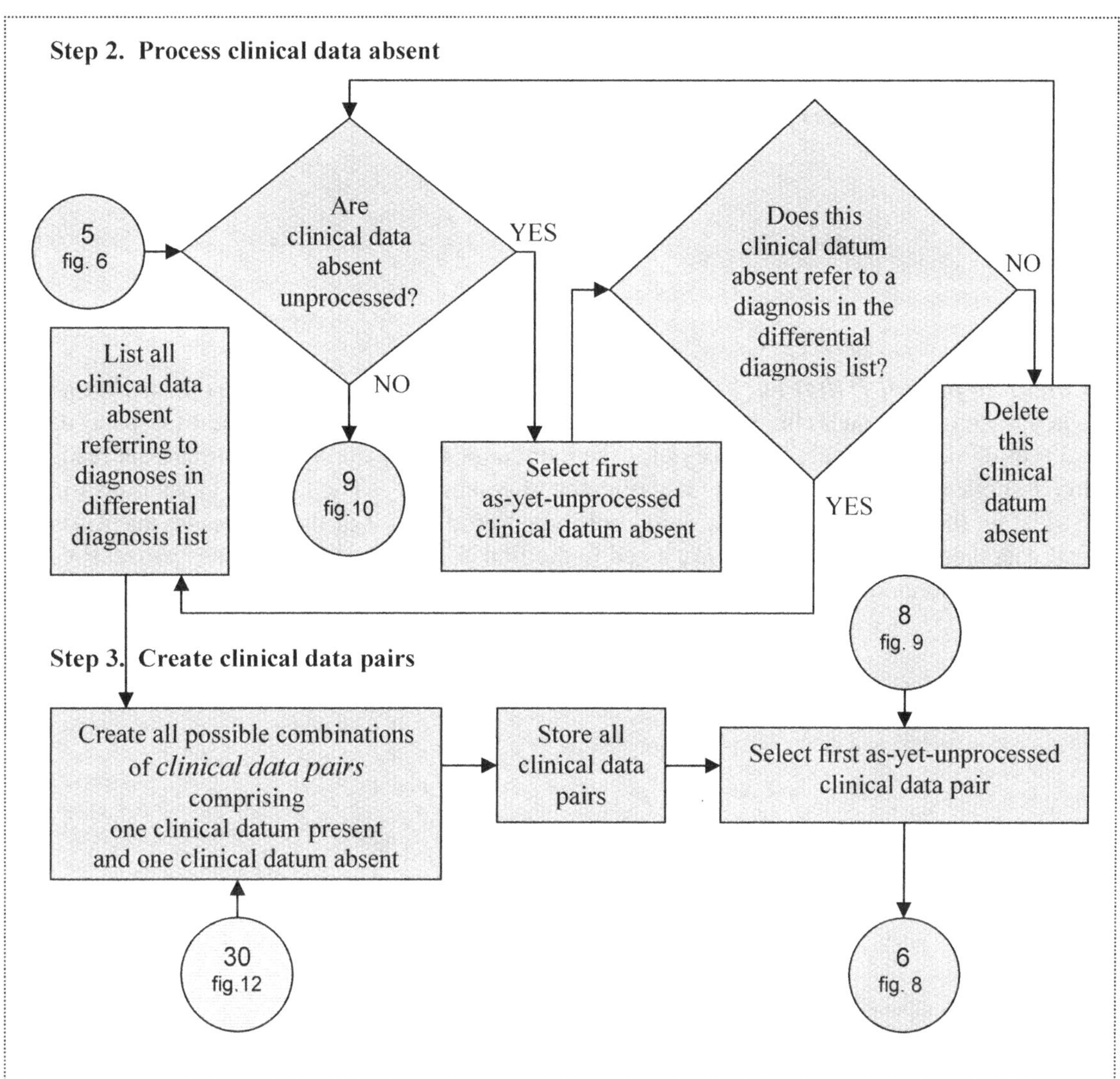

FIGURE 7. CALCULATION OF PROBABILITY OF DIAGNOSES. MINI-MAX PROCEDURE
(continued)

FIGURE 8

Step 4. *Create clinical data pair tables.* Each table is headed by the respective clinical data pair, and lists all differential diagnoses (page 45.)

Step 5. *Calculate partial P that each clinical data pair confers to each differential diagnosis.* First, for each diagnosis in each clinical data pair table, apply equation 7 to PP value of clinical datum present and S of clinical datum absent; this yields the numerator for equation 8. Summate the results of all equation 7 applications; this yields the denominator of equation 8. Then, apply equation 8 to each diagnosis, yielding the partial P values that will contribute to the total P of the respective diagnosis. In each clinical data pair table the diagnoses are listed in the first column, and the resultant partial P values are shown at the last column (page 46.)

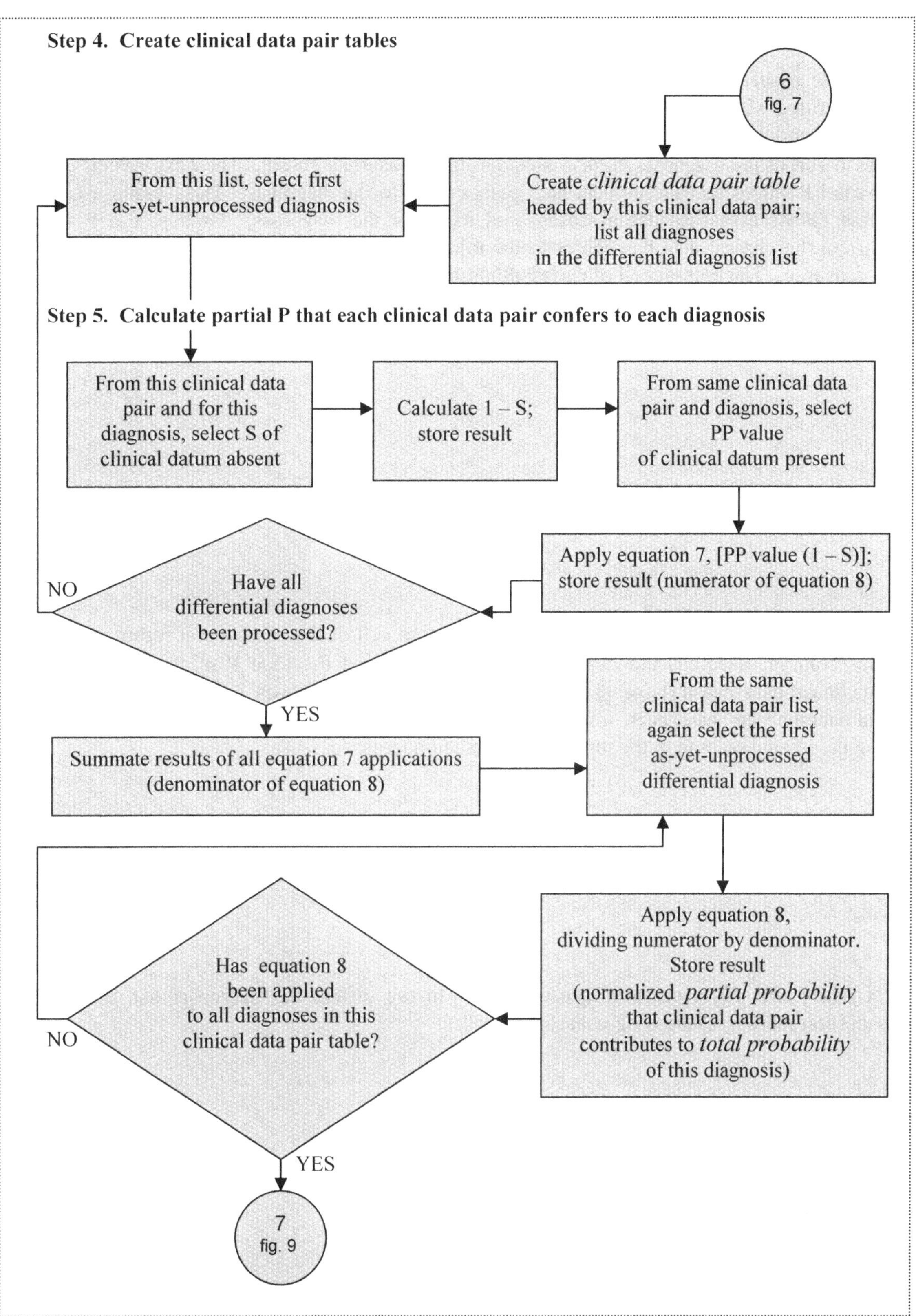

FIGURE 8. CALCULATION OF PROBABILITY OF DIAGNOSES. MINI-MAX PROCEDURE (continued)

FIGURE 9

Step 6. *Create mini-max tables.* For each diagnosis in the differential diagnosis list, create a mini-max table titled with the name of the diagnosis (page 46.). The first column lists all clinical data present. The second column lists their PP values; its bottom cell repeats the greatest of these values, which is the total P of the diagnosis *before* considering clinical data absent. The next several columns show the partial P values that the clinical data pairs confer to the diagnosis. The heading of each of these columns shows a clinical datum absent and its S for the diagnosis. Each partial P value is transferred from the clinical data pair tables to the mini-max table cell where the clinical data present and absent converge. The bottom cell of each column repeats the greatest partial P value in the column. The last column repeats the smallest value in each row.

Step 7. *Determine total P of a diagnosis.* In the bottom cell of the last column repeat the greatest value in this column; it equals the *determining partial P* and the total P of the diagnosis *after* considering clinical data absent (page 48.) Sometimes, total P of a diagnosis, instead of being decreased by a clinical datum absent, as expected, is actually increased. One has the option to preclude this effect by including the second column in the mini-max calculation (page 51.)

Step 8. *Update the differential diagnosis list.* In the differential diagnosis list, update P of diagnoses and sort them by decreasing values (page 50.)

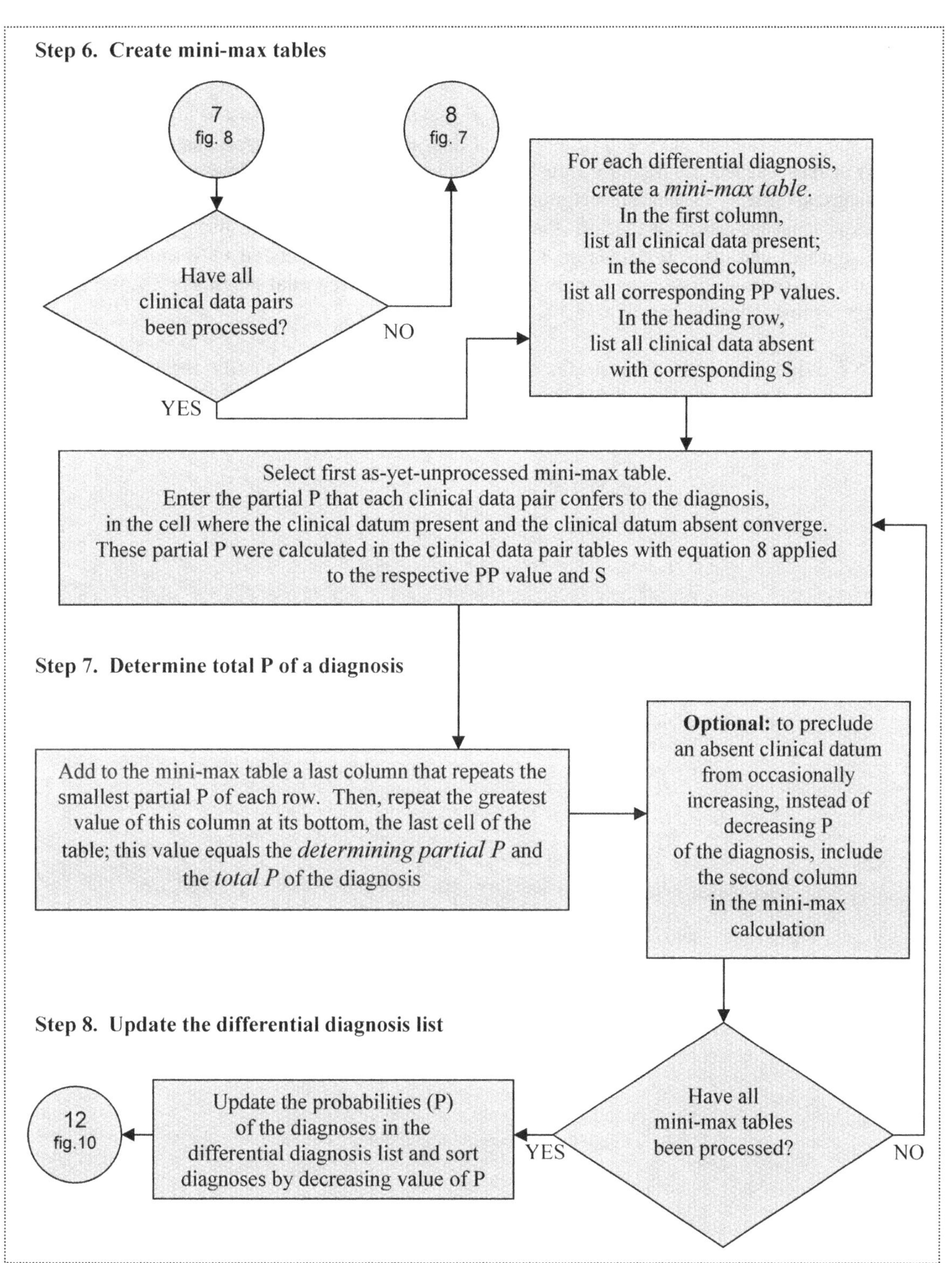

FIGURE 9. CALCULATION OF PROBABILITY OF DIAGNOSES. MINI-MAX PROCEDURE

FIGURE 10. Conclusion of diagnostic quest

Two empiric thresholds are included in the knowledge base: a *confirmation threshold* and a *deletion threshold* (page 87.) Each diagnosis in the differential diagnosis list is checked to ascertain whether its P has reached the confirmation threshold (diagnosis is flagged as final diagnosis and copied into a final diagnoses list) or has reached the deletion threshold (diagnosis is flagged as deleted but retained in the differential diagnosis list.) When all diagnoses in the differential diagnosis list are flagged, the algorithm goes to routines ensuring that no other diagnoses were overlooked; these routines check for risk flagged diagnoses and clinical data (Fig. 17), and clinical entities related with the final diagnoses (Fig. 18). When one or more diagnoses remain unflagged in the differential diagnosis list, the algorithm goes to the next routine (Figs. 11 through 14.)

CONCURRENT DIAGNOSES. Our preferred method selects automatically the concurrent final diagnoses and copies them in the final diagnoses list.

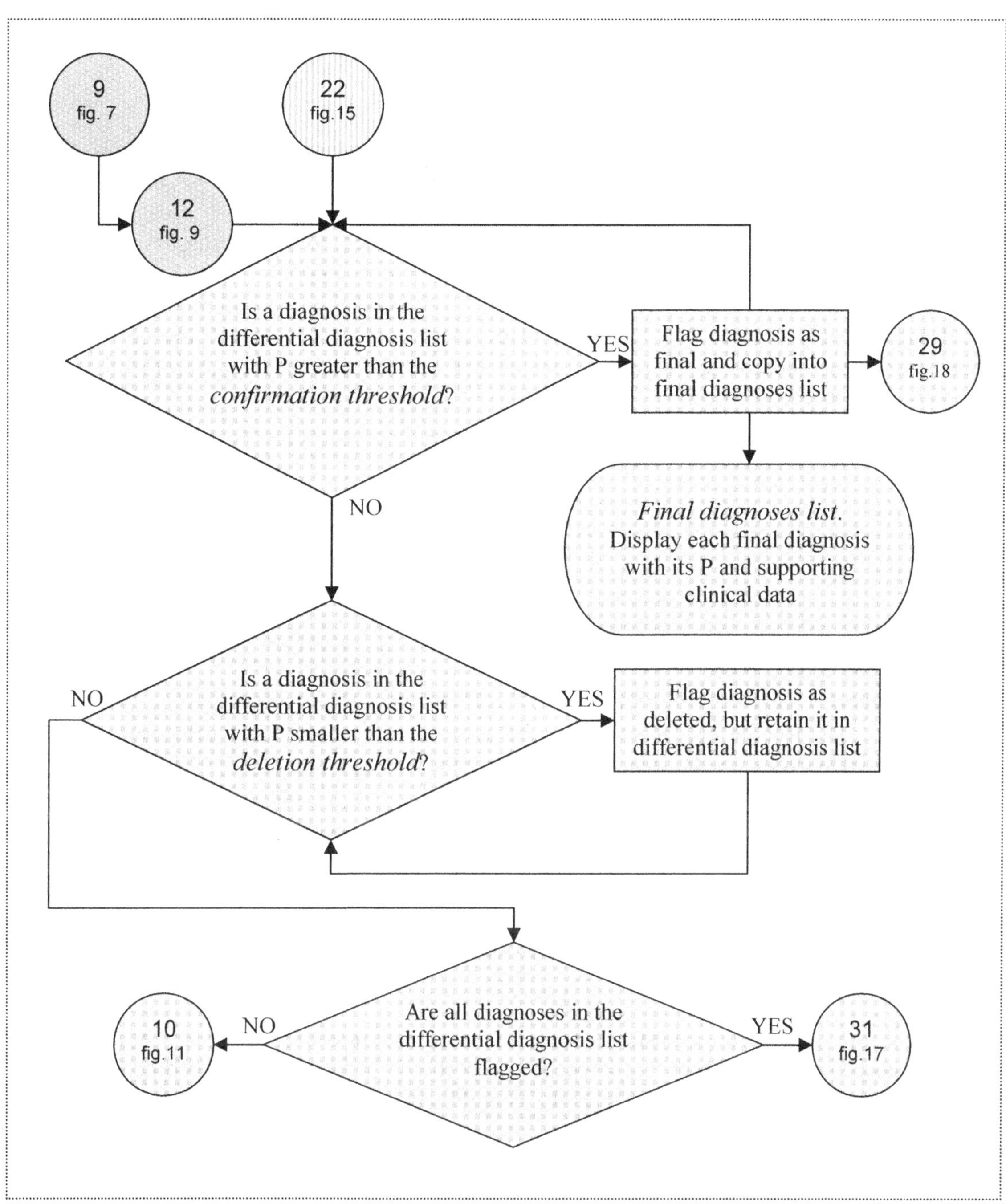

FIGURE 10. CONCLUSION OF DIAGNOSTIC QUEST

FIGURES 11 through 14. Best cost-benefit clinical datum next to investigate

FIGURE 11

Step 1. *Select clinical data not yet investigated in the patient* (page 54.) From the disease models of all diagnoses in the differential diagnosis list, select all remaining clinical data not yet investigated.

Step 2. *Organize clinical data not yet investigated according to cost category, diagnosis, PP value, and S* (page 54.) These clinical data are distributed among four COST categories (no, small, intermediate, and great.) In each cost category, all DIAGNOSES in the differential diagnosis list are repeated and sorted by decreasing P. For each diagnosis and cost category, the corresponding clinical data are sorted by decreasing PP value in one list (PP VALUE LIST), and the *same* clinical data by decreasing S in another list (S LIST.)

Step 3. *Recommend a best cost-benefit clinical datum next to be investigated assuming it present* (page 54.) The routine moves to the lowest as-yet-unprocessed COST category, selects the as-yet-unprocessed DIAGNOSIS with greatest P, and from the corresponding PP VALUE LIST, selects the as-yet-unprocessed clinical datum with the greatest PP value. This PP value then is compared to the PP value of the clinical datum present in the *current* determining clinical data pair. New clinical data with equal or smaller PP value are disregarded because—even if present—they will not change the current P of this diagnosis; accordingly, the routine moves to Step 4. When the PP value of a new clinical datum exceeds the current P of the diagnosis before considering clinical data absent (bottom cell of second column of the mini-max table), the algorithm recommends this best cost-benefit clinical datum.

If the user verifies the recommended best cost-benefit clinical datum as *present*, a new clinical datum list and several new clinical data pairs are created, a new row is inserted in each pertinent mini-max table, and the partial P of the diagnosis assumes the new PP value. The total P of the diagnosis then is recalculated.

If the user verifies the recommended best cost-benefit clinical datum as *absent*, it will be disregarded. Step 3 is iterated until the PP value of a clinical datum in the PP value list does not exceed the current P of the diagnosis.

For simultaneous recommendation of several best cost-benefit clinical data (page 63), first the algorithm assumes that the recommended best cost-benefit clinical datum from the PP value list is virtually present and transfers it to the trichotomy tree (ascending branch) together with the resulting P of the diagnosis (new node.) Then it assumes that the same clinical datum is virtually absent and transfers it to the tree as a horizontal branch; P remains unchanged in the new node.

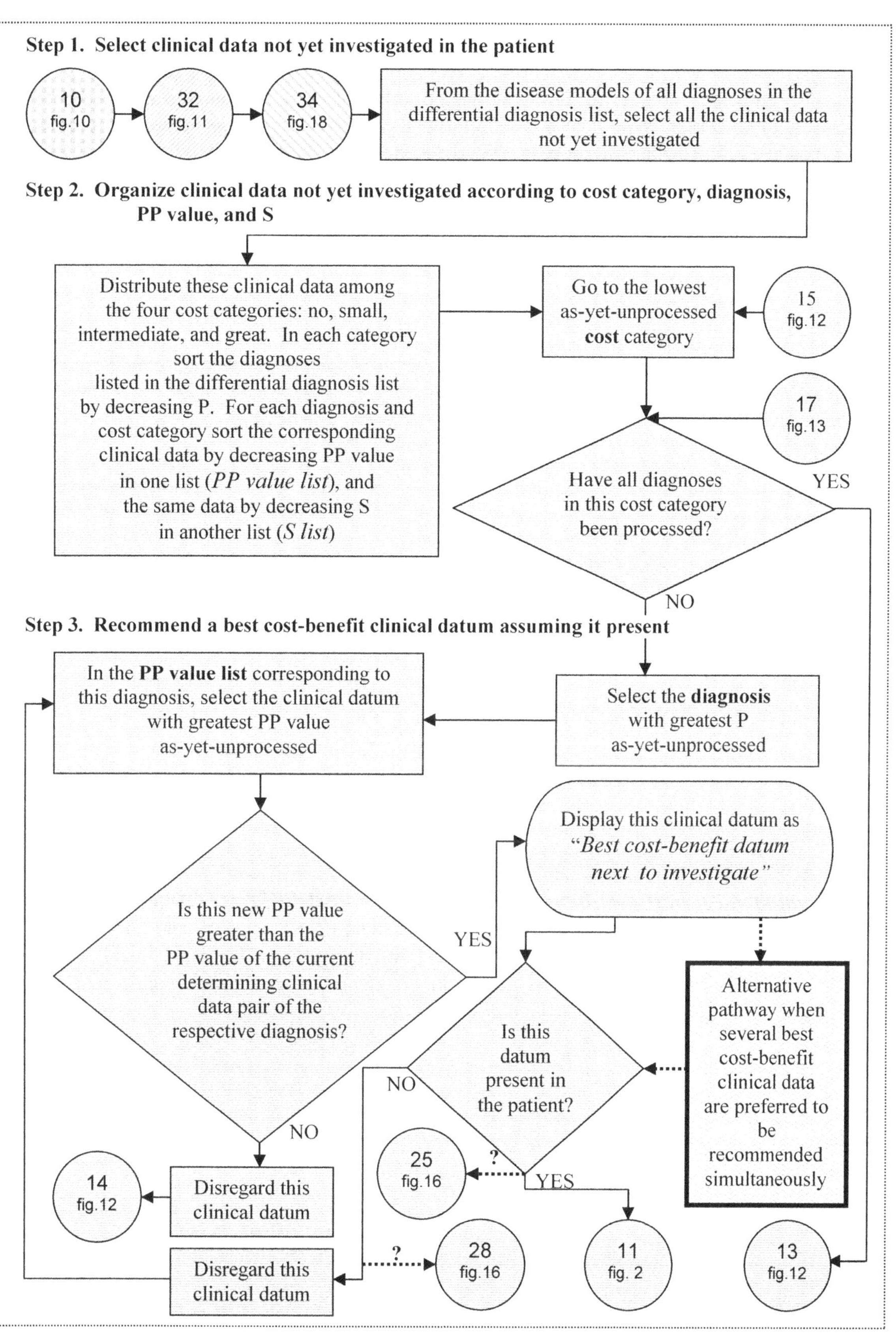

FIGURE 11. BEST COST-BENEFIT CLINICAL DATUM NEXT TO INVESTIGATE (continued)

FIGURE 12

The alternative pathway for several best cost-benefit clinical data recommended simultaneously, bypasses user's authorization request to continue in next greater cost category (page 65) until a final diagnosis is reached or the diagnostic process is deadlocked.

Step 4. ***Recommend a best cost-benefit clinical datum next to be investigated assuming it absent*** (page 58.) From the S LIST corresponding to the same COST category and DIAGNOSIS, the routine selects the as-yet-unprocessed clinical datum with the greatest S; this clinical datum then replaces the existing corresponding datum absent in the *determining clinical data pair*, thereby creating a new clinical data pair.

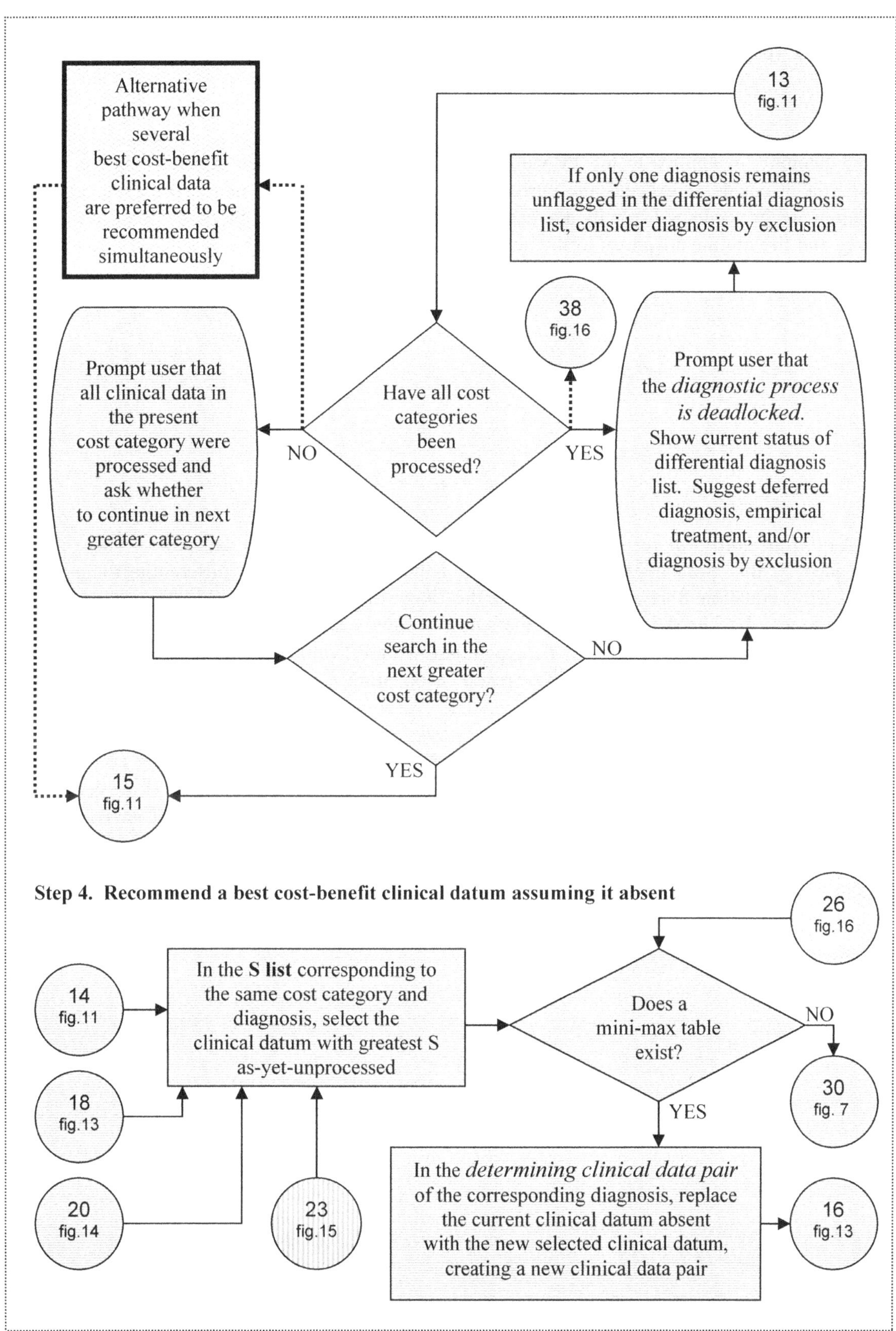

FIGURE 12. BEST COST-BENEFIT CLINICAL DATUM NEXT TO INVESTIGATE (continued)

FIGURES 13 and 14. *3-Step method to predict whether a new clinical datum absent will decrease total P* (page 58.)

FIGURE 13

Step 4.1 Equation 7 is applied to the PP value and S of the newly created clinical data pair. If the resulting partial P equals or exceeds the current total P of the diagnosis, neither *this* nor any *other* clinical datum in the same S list will decrease the total P; accordingly, Steps 4.2 and 4.3 become unnecessary and the routine advances to the next diagnosis. If the resulting P is smaller, the total P of the diagnosis under consideration *may or may not* decrease; proceed to Step 4.2.

Step 4.2 A *clinical data pair table* is created for the newly created clinical data pair of Stage 4.1; this table is headed by this clinical data pair and lists all the diagnoses in the differential diagnosis list (page 60.) Now equation 8 is applied only to the diagnosis being processed; its numerator is as calculated in Step 4.1. The denominator is the sum of terms, each of which is the result of iterating equation 7 applied to the *same* clinical data pair but with PP values and S corresponding to each diagnosis in the clinical data pair table. The result of equation 8 is the normalized partial P for the diagnosis being processed.

If the resulting partial P equals or exceeds the current total P of the diagnosis, the new clinical datum will *not* decrease the total P; Step 4.3 becomes unnecessary for this clinical datum. However, another new clinical datum from the S list, even with a smaller S, still might decrease this total P. To verify the latter, the next new clinical datum from the S list must be tested by Step 4.1 until it fails, at which time the routine moves to the next diagnosis. Conversely, if the resulting partial P is smaller than the current total P of the diagnosis under consideration, the latter *may or may not* decrease. A new column could be created in the mini-max table corresponding to the diagnosis, but only one of its cell can be filled with the calculated partial P. Proceed to Step 4.3.

3-Step method to predict whether a clinical datum absent will decrease P of the corresponding diagnosis

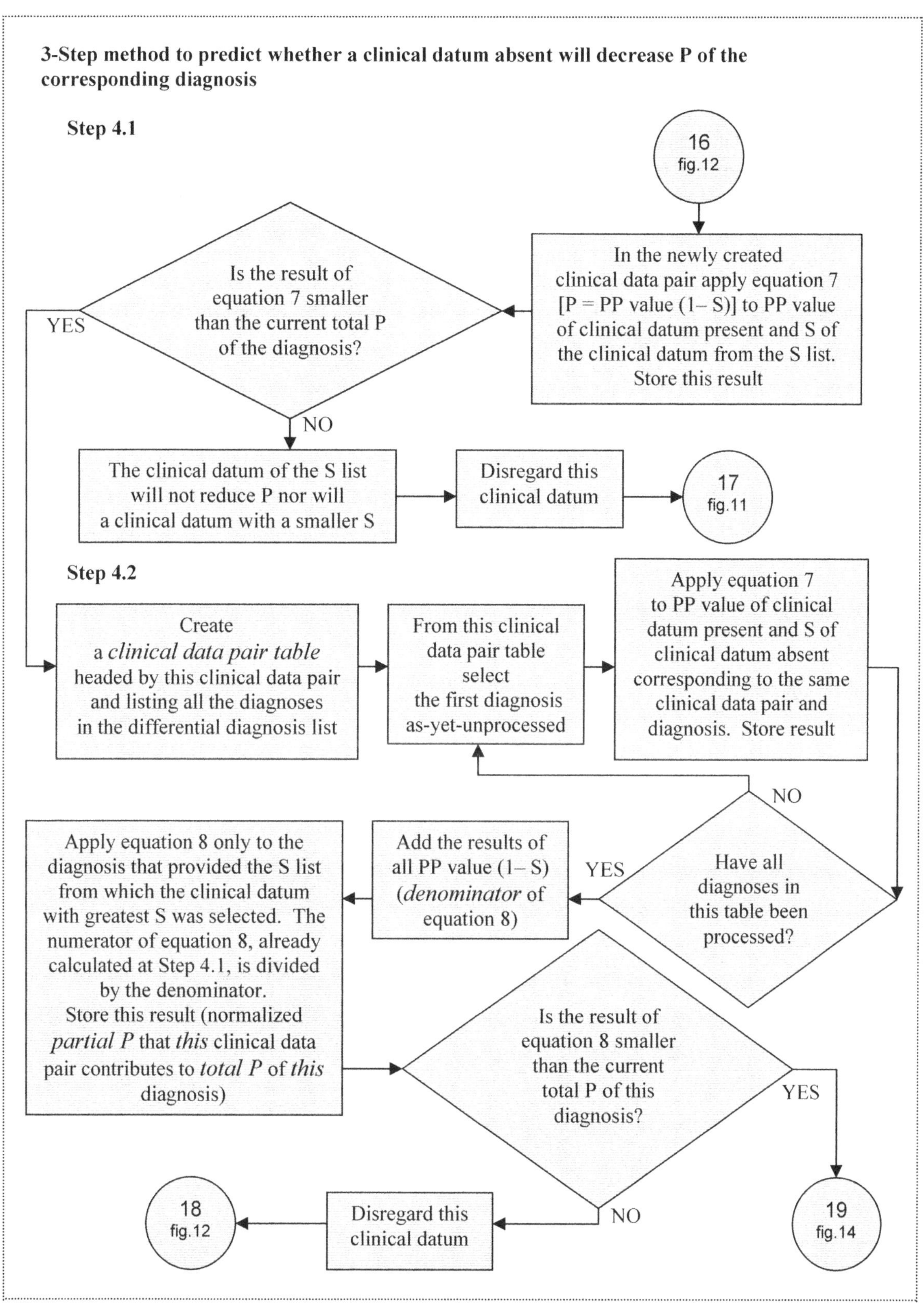

FIGURE 13. BEST COST-BENEFIT CLINICAL DATUM NEXT TO INVESTIGATE (continued)

FIGURE 14

Step 4.3 *All possible* new clinical data pairs and their tables are created, each comprising an existing clinical datum present and the new clinical datum absent (page 60); equation 7 is applied to all diagnoses in all clinical data pairs. Step 4.3 is similar to Step 4.2 except that equation 8 is applied to the diagnosis being processed, but in *all* clinical data pair tables (page 61) instead of in only one. The calculated partial P values that the new clinical data pairs confer to the diagnosis appear in *all* cells of a new column created for the clinical datum absent, in the mini-max table. Total P of the diagnosis is determined. If the new total P is smaller than the existing total P, the new clinical datum from the S list is recommended as the best cost-benefit clinical datum next to investigate; otherwise it is disregarded and the algorithm processes the next clinical datum in the S list. The 3-Step method processes each diagnosis in the differential diagnosis list in a similar way.

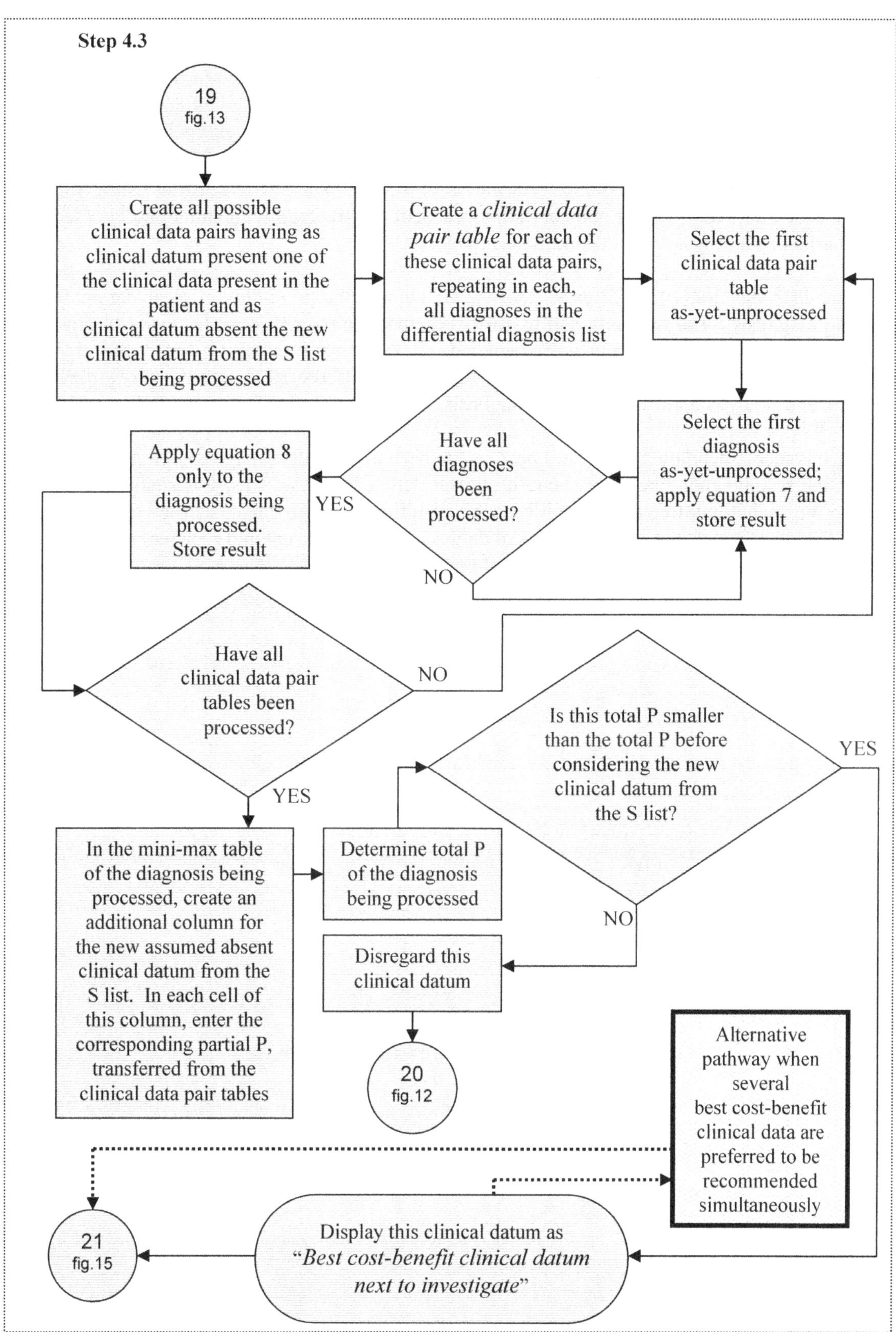

FIGURE 14. BEST COST-BENEFIT CLINICAL DATUM NEXT TO INVESTIGATE

FIGURE 15. Masking

When a best cost-benefit clinical datum is recommended, the user is requested to verify whether it is absent or present. If this clinical datum is present, it is disregarded, no new column is generated in mini-max tables, and the routine returns to the S list, similarly processing the next S clinical datum. If it is absent *and not* flagged with an interaction identifier, the P values in the differential diagnosis list will be updated and sorted by decreasing P; the algorithm goes to Conclusion of Diagnostic Quest (Fig. 10.) If the recommended best cost-benefit clinical datum is absent *and* flagged with an interaction identifier, it might be masked by a drug or concurrent disease (page 88.)

The algorithm lists the drugs and diseases that might change the S of this clinical datum for the corresponding diagnosis. The user is asked to verify whether the patient is medicated with any listed drug, in which case the clinical datum is disregarded. If masking diseases are listed, the algorithm verifies whether these diagnoses have been included in the differential diagnosis list, otherwise it includes them, and if any is confirmed as final diagnosis, the clinical datum is disregarded.

For simultaneous recommendation of several best cost-benefit clinical data (page 63), first the algorithm assumes that the recommended best cost-benefit clinical datum from the S list is virtually present and transfers it to the trichotomy tree (horizontal branch); resulting P of the diagnosis (new node) remains unchanged. Then it assumes that the same clinical datum is virtually absent and transfers it to the tree as a descending branch together with the resulting P of the diagnosis (new node.)

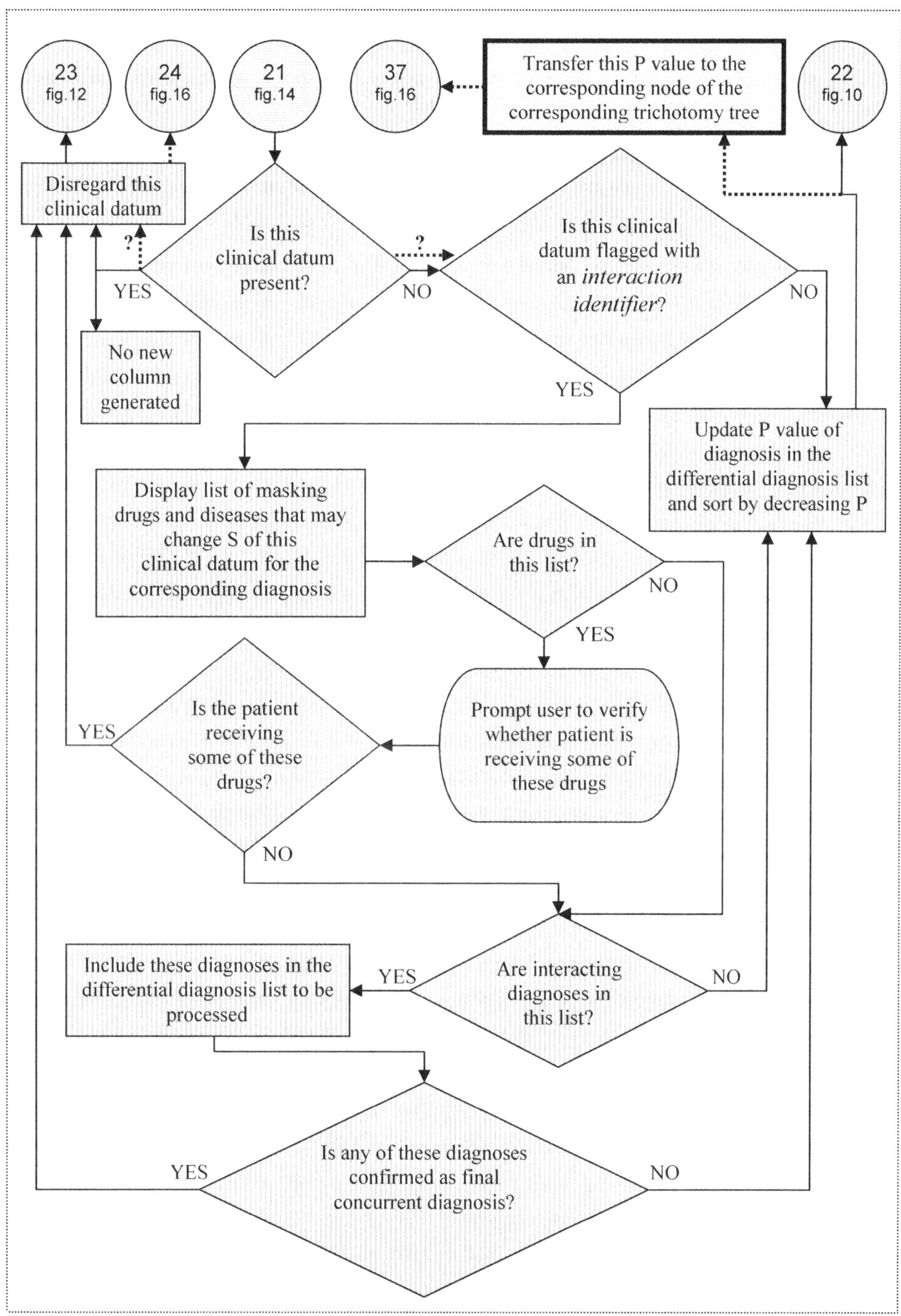

FIGURE 15. MASKING

135

FIGURE 16. Simultaneous recommendation of several best cost-benefit clinical data

A trichotomy tree in progress is created for each diagnosis. Beginning with the current P of the diagnosis, its branches show best cost-benefit clinical data and its nodes show the resulting P of this diagnosis and the cost of obtaining these clinical data (page 63.) Best cost-benefit clinical data recommended by the algorithm are successively assumed virtually present and virtually absent. Ideally, the algorithm explores all possible virtual traversals until maximum or minimum P are attained, or until all available clinical data are exhausted. From all existing trichotomy trees the user must select—according to one or combination of strategies earlier described (page 65)—the best cost-benefit clinical data **set** to be investigated; the selected clinical data, once confirmed present or absent, must be entered in the computer to be processed.

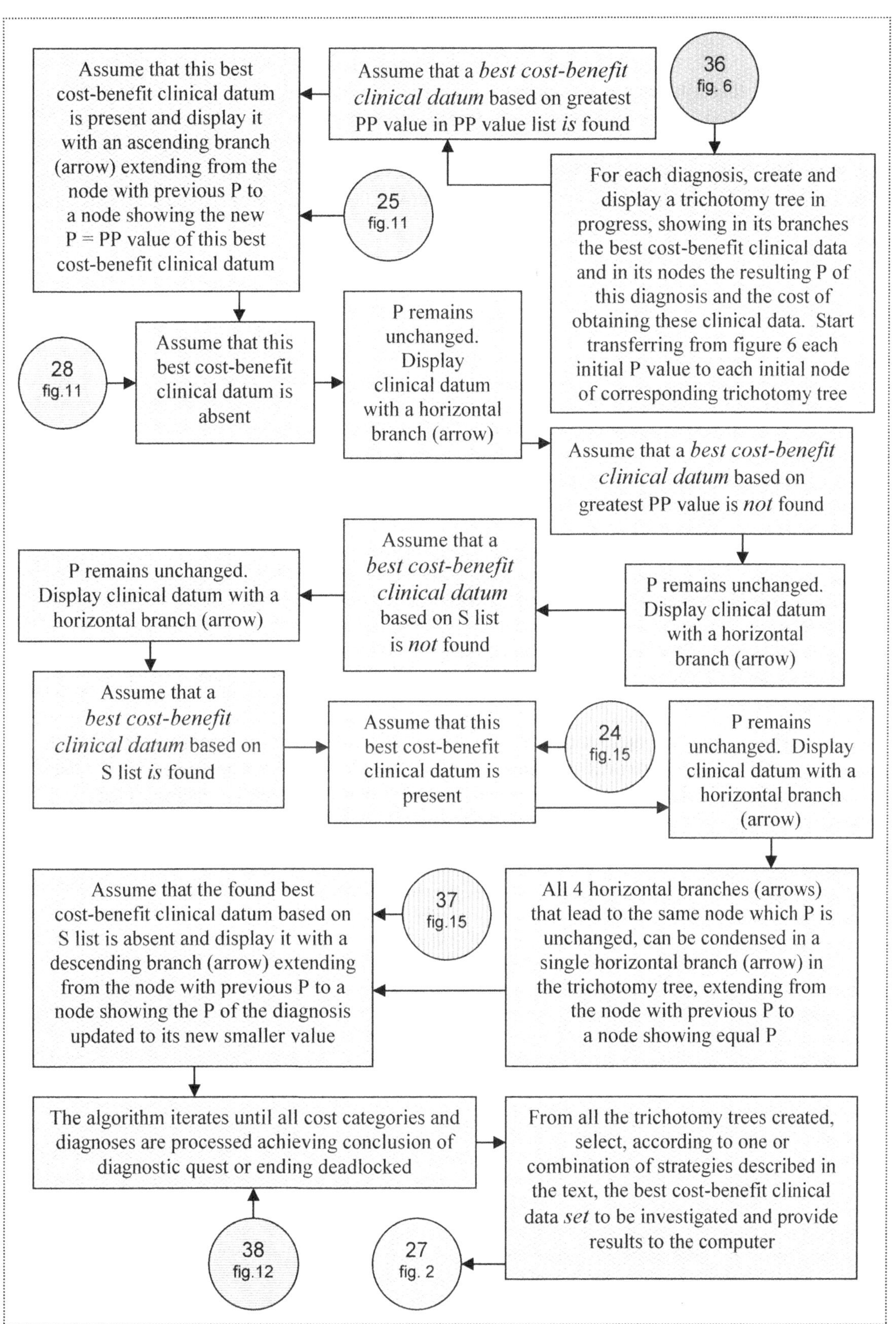

FIGURE 16. SIMULTANEOUS RECOMMENDATION OF SEVERAL BEST COST-BENEFIT CLINAL DATA

FIGURE 17. Safety check for risk flagged diagnoses and clinical data

This routine ensures that all diagnoses flagged with a risk identifier or included in a flagged clinical datum list were included in the differential diagnosis list to be processed for presence or absence (page 89.) This step is superfluous if the preferred all-inclusive method to integrate a differential diagnosis list with all diagnoses in all clinical datum lists is implemented (page 37); in this case the subroutine can directly jump from connector 31 to connector 33 (dashed arrow), bypassing this check.

FIGURE 18. Safety check for related clinical entities

To preclude missing diagnoses, this routine checks for all clinical entities potentially related with each final diagnosis. All complex clinical presentation models in which the final diagnosis is listed are checked, ensuring that all related clinical entities are included in the differential diagnosis list (page 94.)

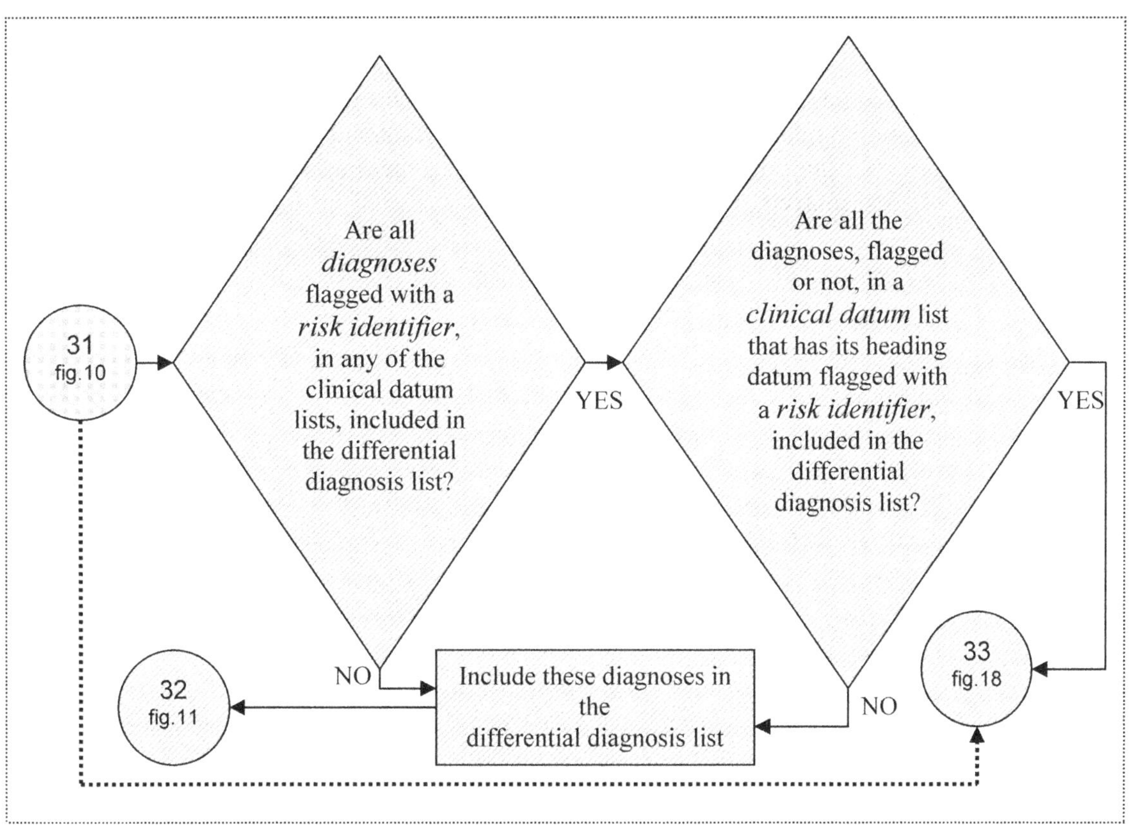

FIGURE 17. SAFETY CHECK FOR RISK FLAGGED DIAGNOSES AND CLINICAL DATA

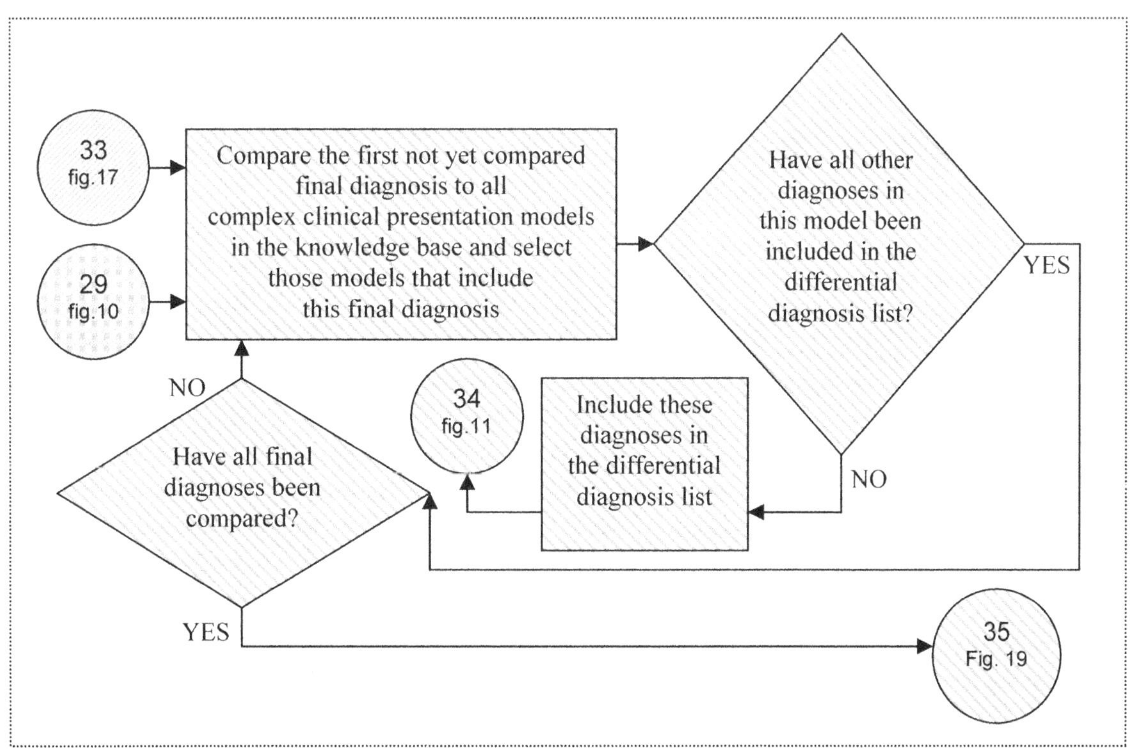

FIGURE 18. SAFETY CHECK FOR RELATED CLINICAL ENTITIES

FIGURE 19. Clinical presentation

When only one final diagnosis is obtained, it is displayed. Concurrent final diagnoses, if included in a complex clinical presentation model, are displayed as a clinical presentation (page 91); otherwise, they are displayed as unrelated final diagnoses. In either case, the message "CONCLUSION OF DIAGNOSTIC QUEST" is displayed.

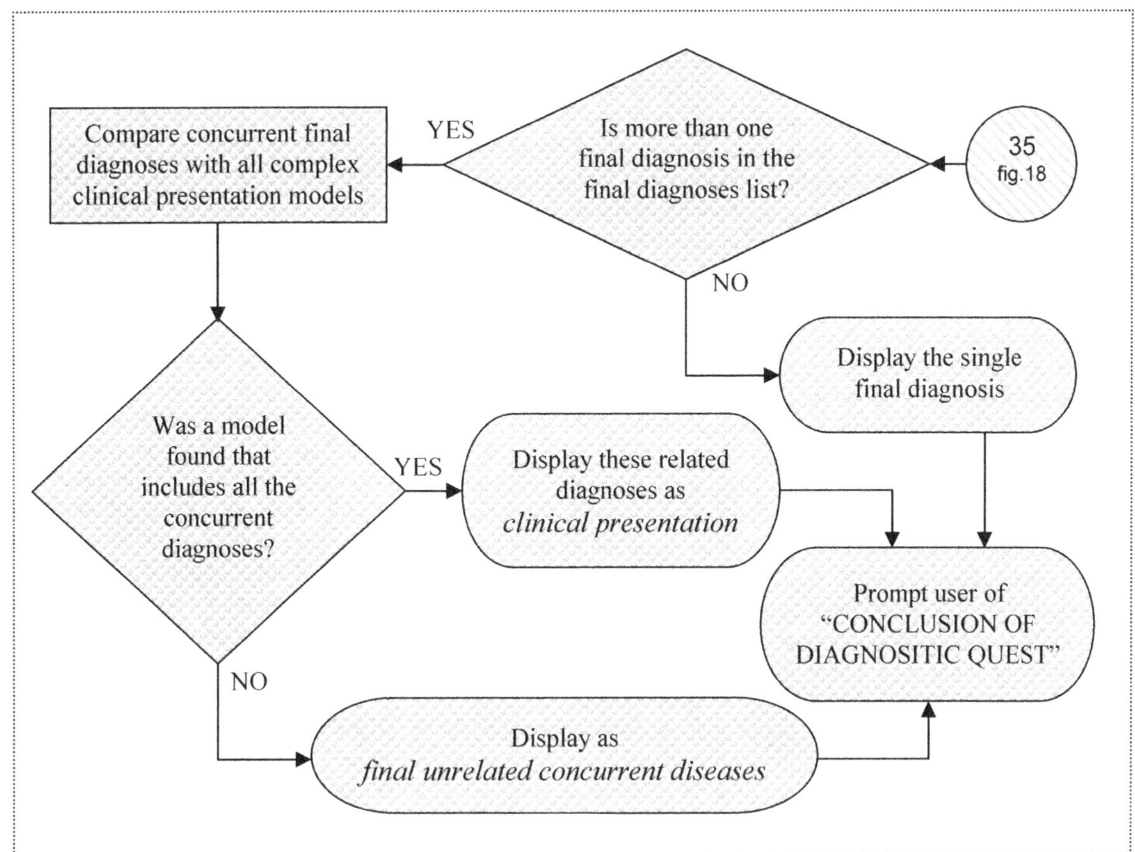

FIGURE 19. CLINICAL PRESENTATION

APPENDIX B: USER INTERFACE

The program should be able to display an initial menu including the following selections among others:

Diagnosis

1. Enter patient's personal information
2. Enter initial clinical data
3. List of entered clinical data (clinical datum lists)
4. Differential diagnosis list
5. Best cost-benefit clinical datum next to investigate
6. Alert when ascending to a greater cost category of best cost-benefit clinical datum next to investigate
7. Enter result, present or absent, of selected best cost-benefit clinical datum
8. Display final diagnosis, concurrent diagnoses, or clinical presentations attained
9. Alert about potential disease or drug interactions
10. Alert about risk flagged clinical data or diseases
11. New case

Medical information

12. Medical information about any disease, including clinical data potentially able to manifest, with corresponding sensitivity, positive predictive value, cost, and risk and interaction identifiers
13. Enter any clinical datum and show which diseases may manifest it, with the corresponding sensitivity and positive predictive value

Update

14. Add new clinical datum
15. Add new disease
16. Add a new clinical presentation
17. Add new risk flag
18. Add new disease or drug interaction
19. Edit disease
20. Edit clinical datum, change its sensitivity, or add new synonym
21. Edit clinical presentation
22. Delete disease
23. Delete clinical datum
24. Delete clinical presentation
25. Delete a risk flag
26. Delete a disease or drug interaction
27. Exit program

These options offer appropriate submenus. One of these submenus could offer the possibility to associate each clinical datum with a number and give the user the choice to enter this clinical datum by name or by number. The latter could save the user to type the entire word for some frequent clinical data. In either case, the computer must confirm the input by displaying the name of the entered datum and ask whether correct or incorrect. When a clinical datum is entered, the submenu will ask whether it is present or absent in the patient.

GLOSSARY

Angina pectoris: chest pain due to coronary artery disease.

Ascites: abnormal accumulation of fluid in the abdominal cavity.

Babinski sign: the extension of big toe with flexion of the other toes when exciting the sole of foot; it is present in some neurologic lesions.

Best cost-benefit clinical datum: is the clinical datum recommended by the algorithm to be investigated in the patient, at each step of the diagnostic process. This clinical datum is expected to have the lowest possible cost and lead most expeditiously to the final diagnosis based on positive predictive value or sensitivity.

Bibasal rales: an abnormal moist sound heard by auscultation, bilaterally, at the lower chest wall, caused by fluid accumulation in the airways at the bases of the lungs.

Bilirubin: principal pigment of bile.

Bruit: an abnormal sound heard during auscultation, usually over a blood vessel.

BUN: Blood Urea Nitrogen.

CBC: Complete Blood Count.

Choledocholithiasis: gallstones in common bile duct.

Choluria: bile pigments in urine that confers it a dark tea or cola color.

Clinical: etymologically relates to a bed; in current usage, it refers to patients. Definition in Webster New International Dictionary, Second Edition: "Investigation of disease in the living subject by observation, as distinguished from controlled experiment." Clinical medicine and clinical lecture are terms mentioned in this dictionary. Accordingly, clinical data, clinical data pair, clinical entity, and clinical presentation are licit terms because they refer to patients. I see no problem in applying by extension the term *clinical* to a model, such as complex clinical presentation model referring to a compilation or inventory of items taken from actual patients (not from experiments.)

Clinical data pair: the combination of a clinical datum present with another absent in the same patient; used to calculate the partial probability that this combination confers to a diagnosis.

Clinical datum (*pl.* DATA): a symptom, sign, or clinical study result that a specific disease may manifest in a given patient.

Clinical datum list: a list headed by a clinical datum and that comprises all potential diagnoses that may manifest this clinical datum.

Clinical entity: a generic term for any element of a *complex clinical presentation*, such as a cause, lesion, syndrome, complication, disease, clinical form, stage, or degree. Clinical data are excluded from this definition because they are elements of a *disease model.*

Clinical form: one of the diverse constellations of clinical data manifested, resulting from a single cause or type of lesion. An *acute* form, displays symptoms that appear suddenly and briefly evolve toward a cure, chronicity, or death (*e.g.*, viral hepatitis.) A *chronic* form has a protracted course (*e.g.*, rheumatoid arthritis.) Some forms depend on *lesion localization* (*e.g.*, pulmonary, intestinal, renal, or genital tuberculosis.) Other forms depend on *lesion characteristics* (*e.g.*, fibrotic, caseous, miliary, or cavitary tuberculosis.) *Each clinical form has its own disease model.*

Competing diagnoses: diagnoses included in a differential diagnosis list, which compete for the greatest probability (P), ultimately becoming a final diagnosis or being ruled out.

Complex clinical presentation: two or more final diagnoses are needed to account for all manifested clinical data. For example, coronary artery disease, acute myocardial infarction, congestive heart failure, shock, *and* thromboembolism in a single patient.

Complex clinical presentation model: a list of all diseases or clinical entities that are potentially related by pathophysiologic links or statistical correlations.

Complication: a secondary disease or medical condition linked to a primary disease. Typically, a lesion of the primary disease conditions the action of an added cause producing the complication. Example of an added cause is an ingrown nail (primary cause) that provokes a wound (primary lesion), which allows the entry of bacteria (secondary or added cause) provoking infection (secondary disease.)

Concurrent diagnoses or diseases: more than one disease affecting a specific patient.

Determining clinical data pair: the clinical data pair that comprises the clinical datum *present* with the PP value that most effectively *increases* the P of a diagnosis and the clinical datum *absent* with the S that most effectively *reduces* the P of a diagnosis. This PP value has the greatest rule-in effect; this S has the greatest rule-out effect. The determining clinical data pair is so named because applying equation 8 to its PP value and S value yields the determining partial P.

Determining partial P: the partial P that determines and equals the total P of the corresponding diagnosis. Transferred to the mini-max table, it is at once the *smallest value in its row* and the *greatest value in its column* and occupies the cell to which converge the clinical datum present and the clinical datum absent of the determining clinical data pair.

Diabetes insipidus: a disease characterized by excessive thirst, excessive urination, and diluted urine, caused by a decreased secretion or impaired response to antidiuretic hormone, caused by a neurohypophyseal or kidney lesion.

Diagnosis: the identification of an abnormal condition that afflicts a patient, based on manifested clinical data.

Disease: a condition in which physicochemical parameter values are out of range and health qualities, such as well-being, harmony in all body functions, and the ability to establish and fulfill goals in life, are altered; in other words, a malfunctioning of the organism. It typically leads to structural changes or lesions.

Disease Model: An abstract concept that combines all possible clinical data that a disease manifests in a large population of patients. It includes the sensitivity, positive predictive value, cost, and—if pertinent—risk identifier and masking susceptibility of clinical data. A disease model may also include or offer links to other medical concepts such as etiology, pathogenesis, pathology, pathophysiology, complications, prognosis, and treatment. Disease models are stored in the computer knowledge base.

Dyspnea: difficulty to breathe; shortness of breath.

ECG: ElectroCardioGram.

Entity: see clinical entity.

DNA: DeoxyriboNucleic Acid; a nucleic acid, essence of the genetic code of living beings.

ERCP: Endoscopic Retrograde CholangioPancreatography. A combined endoscopic and radiographic procedure that enables instillation of a contrast medium into the bile and pancreatic ducts so as to visualize these anatomical parts.

ESR: Erythrocyte Sedimentation Rate.

Etiology: the study of the causes of diseases; sometimes used as synonym of the cause (*e.g.*, the etiology of tuberculosis is *Mycobacterium tuberculosis*.)

Fremitus: a palpable vibration sensed by the flat hand placed over a body area, usually the chest wall.

Fundoscopy: the examination of the interior of the eye, especially the retina, with an ophthalmoscope.

Gallop rhythm: a cadence of three heart sounds resembling the sound of a galloping horse, that is characteristic of congestive heart failure, among other medical conditions.

Hemoptysis: blood expectorated from the respiratory tract.

Hepatomegaly: liver enlargement.

Heuristic: a problem-solving method that simplifies and shortens a computer process, based on experience, rules of thumb, insight, or intuition, as opposed to an algorithm that involves **exhaustive** search, collection, and processing of information.

Hypochondriasis: mental disorder characterized by an abnormal concern of being afflicted by a serious organic disease, based on misinterpretation of minor abnormalities or even normal sensations.

Iatrogenic: disorder or complication produced by a treatment or a physician.

Laparoscopy: the examination of the abdominal cavity through a small incision of the abdominal wall using an instrument called a laparoscope.

Laparotomy: an incision through the abdominal wall providing a direct view of the abdominal organs.

Menarche: the first appearance of menstruation.

Mini-max procedure: combines positive predictive value (PP value) of clinical data present (favoring a diagnosis) and sensitivity (S) of clinical data absent (disfavoring a diagnosis), to calculate the resulting probability (P) of a diagnosis.

Mini-max table: a table that registers the partial probabilities that clinical data pairs confer to a diagnosis and integrates these partial probabilities into the total probability of the diagnosis.

MRI: Magnetic Resonance Imaging: an imaging technique that does not involve X-rays and enables visualizing of internal organs of a body.

***Mycobacterium tuberculosis*:** the bacillus that causes tuberculosis.

Murmur: a blowing, whistling, or rolling sound heard on auscultation over the heart or a blood vessel.

Nash equilibrium: in game theory, a pair of distributions P and Q, such that given P it is minimized by Q, and given Q it is maximized by P. In other words, when a player correctly predicts his o her opponent strategy, and plays an optimal response to these predictions, the strategy results in Nash equilibrium.

Negative predictive value (NP value): conditional probability of *disease absent* given a clinical datum absent. 1–NP value defines an index that represents the *strength with which a clinical datum absent disfavors a specific diagnosis*.

Normalization: (1) Transformation of a set of values into another set of values that sum 1, maintaining the original proportion among them—ascribing percentage values. (2) Transformation of tree or network association of data into tables without loss of information about the associations between these data.

NP value: see Negative predictive value.

Ontology: the description of concepts, their characteristics and relationships in a specific domain or instantiation, then abstracted with the intention to reuse them applied to a different domain.

Otoscopy: the examination of the ear canal and tympanic membrane with an otoscope.

Pathogenesis: the mechanism by which a cause produces a lesion.

Pathognomonic: denotes a clinical datum that is characteristic and exclusive for a specific disease or diagnosis; the PP value of this clinical datum for this diagnosis equals 1.

Pathology: the study of lesions produced by a disease.

Pathophysiology: the mechanism by which a lesion causes abnormal function, or the discipline that studies such mechanisms.

Photophobia: light intolerance.

Pneumothorax: the presence of air or gas in the pleural space.

Polydipsia: excessive thirst.

Polyuria: excessive production of urine.

Positive predictive value (PP value): the probability of a disease in a patient that manifests a clinical datum. The greater the PP value, the more a clinical datum *present* supports a diagnosis.

PSA: Prostate Specific Antigen; blood levels increase with prostate cancer.

PP value: see Positive predictive value.

PP value list: clinical data not yet investigated for presence or absence in the patient, and sorted by decreasing positive predictive value (PP value) in each cost category and for each diagnosis in the differential diagnosis list.

Rebound tenderness: pain elicited by sudden release of localized compression of the abdominal wall over an acutely inflamed organ, *e.g.*, appendicitis.

Red herring: anything that diverts attention from the main question.

ROC (Receiver Operating Characteristic) curve: a curve of a function in a two-dimensional system of rectangular coordinates that represents a problem in which no clear limit exists between normal and abnormal or true and false, but instead a gray zone. The operator, in this case the physician, must select a point (cutoff point) of this curve that enables his best decision-making. Moving the cutoff point increases the accuracy of the result but involves greater cost; similarly, it will confer greater sensitivity to a test (detect more cases of a disease) but decreases specificity (result in more false positives.)

Romberg sign: The loss of balance that occurs when the eyes are closed and the feet are placed together, as observed in certain neurologic diseases.

S: see Sensitivity.

S list: clinical data not yet investigated for presence or absence in the patient, and sorted by decreasing sensitivity (S) in each cost category and for each diagnosis in the differential diagnosis list.

Sensitivity (S) of a clinical datum: the fraction of patients with a given disease who manifest the clinical datum. *In our algorithm,* the greater the S value of a clinical datum *absent*, the less likely the corresponding diagnosis.

Sign: objective clue of disease that a clinician detects during steps of the physical examination: inspection (observing the patient), palpation (feeling the shape, temperature, consistency, tenderness of organs), percussion (tapping the surface of the body and listening to the elicited sound), auscultation (listening to sounds produced by organs), and other maneuvers.

Specificity of a clinical datum: the fraction of patients without a disease who do not manifest the clinical datum. Our algorithm does not use specificity.

Splenomegaly: enlargement of the spleen.

Symptom: abnormal feeling manifested by a patient.

Syndrome: a meaningful association of clinical data relating to a common originating cause or lesion, via corresponding pathophysiologic mechanisms.

Thrombosis: an abnormal blood clot formation inside the heart or a blood vessel.

Thromboembolism: a thrombosis complicated by migration of a clot from its site of origin to a downstream site where it becomes lodged, obstructing the vessel (this process is called embolism.)

TIBC: Total Iron Binding Capacity.

Trophism: nutritional status of an organ or tissue.

TSH: Thyroid Stimulating Hormone.

REFERENCES

[1] NOY NF and MUSEN MA. Ontology Versioning as an Element of an Ontology-Management Framework. Stanford Medical Informatics, Stanford University, 251 Campus Drive, Stanford, CA 94305, USA. SMI-2003-0961. March 31, 2003

[2] GENNARI J, MUSEN MA, FERGERSON RW, GROSSO WE, CRUBEZY M, ERIKSSON H, NOY NF, TU SW: The Evolution of Protégé: An Environment for Knowledge-Based Systems Development. 2002. SMI-2002-0943

[3] CHAKRAVARTY S and SHAHAR Y. Acquisition and Analysis of Periodic Patterns in Time-Oriented Clinical Data. 2000. SMI-2000-0822

[4] CHAKRAVARTY S and SHAHAR Y. A Constraint-Based Specification of Periodic Patterns in Time-Oriented Data. Sixth International Workshop on Temporal Representation and Reasoning (TIME-99), Orlando, FL, 29-40. 1999. SMI-1999-0766

[5] ALTMAN RB. AI in Medicine: The Spectrum of Challenges from Managed Care to Molecular Medicine. AI Magazine 20(3):67-77, 1999. SMI-1999-0770

[6] GREENS RA, PELEG M, BOSWALA AA, TU S, PATEL VL, and SHORTLIFFE EH. Sharable Computer-Based Clinical Practice Guidelines: Rationale, Obstacles, Approaches, and Prospects. Medinfo, London, UK, 2001. SMI-2001-0860

[7] TU SW et al: Modeling Guidelines for Integration into Clinical Workflow. Department of Medicine, Stanford University School of Medicine, Stanford, CA, USA. SMI-2003-0970

[8] SHORTLIFFE EH. The Next Generation Internet and Health Care: A Civics Lesson for the Informatics Community. In C.G. Chute, Ed., 1998 AMIA Annual Symposium, Orlando, FL, 8-14. 1998. SMI-98-0730

[9] GINI RA and FEDER C. Informatica Clinica: Presente y Futuro. La Semana Medica (Argentina) 157: 113-128, 1980

[10] ILIAD® 4.5 Diagnostic and Reference Tool for Physicians and Medical Professionals. User Guide. 1998

[11] SHWE M, MIDDLETON B, HECKERMAN D, HENRION M, HORVITZ E, LEHMANN H, & COOPER G. Probabilistic Diagnosis Using a Reformulation of the INTERNIST-1/QMR Knowledge Base I. The Probabilistic Model and Inference Algorithms. Methods of Information in Medicine, 30(4):241-255, 1991. SMI-90-0296

[12] MIDDLETON B, SHWE M, HECKERMAN D, HENRION M, HORVITZ E, LEHMANN H, & COOPER G: Probabilistic Diagnosis using a reformulation of the INTERNIST-1/QMR Knowledge Base II. Evaluation of Diagnostic Performance. Section on Medical Informatics Technical report SMI-90-0329, Stanford University, 1990

[13] MYERS JD, POPLE HE, and MILLER RA. INTERNIST: Can Artificial Intelligence Help? In: Connelly, Benson, Burke, Fenderson, eds. Clinical Decisions and Laboratory Use. Minneapolis: University of Minnesota Press, 1982: 251-269

[14] MILLER RA, POPLE HE, and MYERS JD. INTERNIST-I, An Experimental Computer-Based Diagnostic Consultant for General Internal Medicine. The New England Journal of Medicine, 1982: 468-476

[15] LUDWIG DW. INFERNET – A Computer-Based System for Modeling Medical Knowledge and Clinical Inference. Proceedings of the Fifth Annual Symposium on Computer Applications in Medical Care: 243-249, November 1981

[16] SZOLOVITS P and PAUKER SG. Categorical and Probabilistic Reasoning in Medical Diagnosis. Artificial Intelligence. 11: 115-144, 1978

[17] PERLROTH MG, and WEILAND DJ. Fifty Diseases: Fifty Diagnoses. Year Book Medical Publishers, 1981

[18] WEISS S, KULIKOWSKI CA, and SAFIR A. Glaucoma Consultation by Computer. Comput. Biol. Med. 8: 25-40, 1978

[19] BLEICH HL. Computer-Based Consultation: Electrolyte and Acid-Base Disorders. The American Journal of Medicine 53: 285-291, November 1972

[20] DE DOMBAL FT, LEAPER DJ, STANILAND JR, McCANN AP, and HORROCKS JC. Computer-Aided Diagnosis of Acute Abdominal Pain. British Medical Journal 2: 9-13, 1972

[21] LEDLEY RS and LUSTED LB. Reasoning Foundations of Medical Diagnosis. Science, 130 (9): 9-21, July 3, 1959

[22] LUSTED LB. Introduction to Medical Decision Making. Springfield, Illinois, Charles C Thomas, 1968

[23] LUSTED LB. Twenty Years of Medical Decision Making Studies. CH1480-3/79/0000-0004$00.75. 1979 IEEE

[24] POPLE HE. Heuristic Methods for Imposing Structure on Ill-structured Problems: The Structuring of Medical Diagnosis. In: Szolovits P, ed. Artificial Intelligence in Medicine, AAAS Symposium Series, Boulder, Colorado: West-view Press, 1982: 119-185

[25] BLOIS MS, TUTTLE MS, and SHERERTZ DD. RECONSIDER: A Program for Generating Differential Diagnoses. IEEE: 263-268, 1981

[26] HENRION M, PRADHAN M, DEL FAVERO B, HUANG K, and O'RORKE P: Why is diagnosis using belief networks insensitive to imprecision in probabilities? Twelfth Conference on Uncertainty in Artificial Intelligence, Portland, OR, 446-454. 1996. SMI-96-0637

[27] MARTIN J: Computer Data-Base Organization. Prentice-Hall, Inc., Englewood Cliffs, New Jersey, 1977

[28] POPLE HE, MYERS JD, and MILLER RA: Dialog: A Model of Diagnostic Logic for Internal Medicine. Fourth International Joint Conference on Artificial Intelligence. Tbilisi, Georgia, URRS, 3-8 September 1975, Volume Two. 1975: 848-855

[29] SHORTLIFE EH. Computer-Based Medical Consultations: MYCIN. American Elsevier Publishing Company, 1976

CHAKRAVARTY S, SHAHAR Y: A Constraint-Based Specification of Periodic Patterns in Time-Oriented Data. Sixth International Workshop on Temporal Representation and Reasoning (TIME-99), Orlando, FL, 29-40. 1999. SMI-1999-0766

ESHELMAN L, EHRET D, McDERMOTT JP, and TAN M (1987.) MOLE: A Tenacious Knowledge Acquisition Tool. International Journal of Man-Machine Studies, 26: 41-54

GORRY GA, KASSIRER JP, ESSIG A, and SCHWARTZ WB. Decision Analysis as the Basis for Computer-Aided Management of Acute Renal Failure. The American Journal of Medicine 55: 473-484, 1973

GORRY GA, PAUKER SG, and SCHWARTZ WB. The Diagnostic Importance of the Normal Finding. The new England Journal of Medicine 486-489, March 2, 1978

HUANG K, HENRION M: Efficient Search-Based Inference for Noisy-OR Belief Networks: Top Epsilon. Proceedings of the Twelfth Conference of Uncertainty in Artificial Intelligence, 325-331. Aug 1996, Portland, OR. SMI-96-0640

JAAKKOLA TS, JORDAN MI: Variational Probabilistic Inference and the QMR-DT Network. Sun May 9, 16:22:01 PDT 1999

MUSEN MA: Modeling for Decision Support. Section on Medical Informatics. Stanford University School of Medicine. Stanford, CA 94305-5479. SMI-98-0739

MUSSEN MA, GENNARI JH, and WONG WW: A Rational Reconstruction of INTERNIST-I Using PROTÉGÉ-II. Nineteenth Annual Symposium on Computer Applications in Medial Care. New Orleans, LA, 289-293. 1995. SMI-95-0574

PATRICK EA: Decision Analysis in Medicine: Methods and Applications. CRC Press, West Palm Beach, FL, 1979

PRADHAN M, DAGUM P: Optimal Monte Carlo Estimation of Belief Network Inference. Proceedings of the Twelfth Conference of Uncertainty in Artificial Intelligence, 446-453. Aug 1996, Portland, OR. SMI-96-0638

VAN BEMMEL JH, MUSSEN MA (eds): Medical Informatics. Springer, 1997

WEINSTEIN MC and FINEBERG HV: Clinical Decision Analysis. W. B. Saunders Company, 1980

INDEX

Made in the USA
Monee, IL
07 July 2026

56550065R00096